Master of Public Health Competencies

A CASE STUDY APPROACH

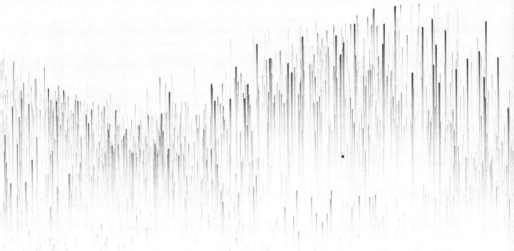

Edited by:

Anthony J. Santella, DrPH, MPH, MCHES
Hofstra University

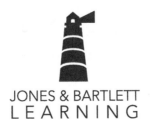

JONES & BARTLETT
LEARNING

World Headquarters
Jones & Bartlett Learning
5 Wall Street
Burlington, MA 01803
978-443-5000
info@jblearning.com
www.jblearning.com

Jones & Bartlett Learning books and products are available through most bookstores and online booksellers. To contact Jones & Bartlett Learning directly, call 800-832-0034, fax 978-443-8000, or visit our website, www.jblearning.com.

Substantial discounts on bulk quantities of Jones & Bartlett Learning publications are available to corporations, professional associations, and other qualified organizations. For details and specific discount information, contact the special sales department at Jones & Bartlett Learning via the above contact information or send an email to specialsales@jblearning.com.

Copyright © 2020 by Jones & Bartlett Learning, LLC, an Ascend Learning Company

All rights reserved. No part of the material protected by this copyright may be reproduced or utilized in any form, electronic or mechanical, including photocopying, recording, or by any information storage and retrieval system, without written permission from the copyright owner.

The content, statements, views, and opinions herein are the sole expression of the respective authors and not that of Jones & Bartlett Learning, LLC. Reference herein to any specific commercial product, process, or service by trade name, trademark, manufacturer, or otherwise does not constitute or imply its endorsement or recommendation by Jones & Bartlett Learning, LLC and such reference shall not be used for advertising or product endorsement purposes. All trademarks displayed are the trademarks of the parties noted herein. *Master of Public Health Competencies: A Case Study Approach* is an independent publication and has not been authorized, sponsored, or otherwise approved by the owners of the trademarks or service marks referenced in this product.

There may be images in this book that feature models; these models do not necessarily endorse, represent, or participate in the activities represented in the images. Any screenshots in this product are for educational and instructive purposes only. Any individuals and scenarios featured in the case studies throughout this product may be real or fictitious, but are used for instructional purposes only.

This publication is designed to provide accurate and authoritative information in regard to the Subject Matter covered. It is sold with the understanding that the publisher is not engaged in rendering legal, accounting, or other professional service. If legal advice or other expert assistance is required, the service of a competent professional person should be sought.

Production Credits
VP, Product Management: Amanda Martin
Director of Product Management: Cathy Esperti
Product Manager: Sophie Fleck Teague
Product Specialist: Carter McAlister
Project Specialist: Kelly Sylvester
Digital Products Manager: Jordan McKenzie
Digital Project Specialist: Angela Dooley
Senior Marketing Manager: Susanne Walker
Manufacturing and Inventory Control
   Supervisor: Amy Bacus

Composition: codeMantra U.S. LLC
Cover Design: Kristin E. Parker
Rights & Media Specialist: Maria Leon Maimone
Media Development Editor: Shannon Sheehan
Cover Image (Title Page, Section Opener,
   Chapter Opener): © royyimzy/Getty Images
Printing and Binding: McNaughton & Gunn
Cover Printing: McNaughton & Gunn

Library of Congress Cataloging-in-Publication Data
Names: Santella, Anthony J., editor.
Title: Master of public health competencies: a case studies approach /
edited by Anthony J. Santella, DrPH, MPH, MCHES.
Description: Burlington, Massachusetts: Jones & Bartlett Learning, [2020] | Includes bibliographical references.
Identifiers: LCCN 2018059554 | ISBN 9781284166323 (paperback)
Subjects: LCSH: Public health personnel—Education. | Public health—Study and teaching.
Classification: LCC RA440.8 .M37 2020 | DDC 362.1076—dc23
LC record available at https://lccn.loc.gov/2018059554

6048

Printed in the United States of America
25 24 23 22 21   10 9 8 7 6 5 4 3 2

© royyimzy/Getty Images

Contents

Contributors

▶ Chapter 1

Ajay Anand Myneni, PhD, MBBS, MPH
Research Scientist
Department of Epidemiology and
 Environmental Health
School of Public Health and Health
 Professions
University at Buffalo
Buffalo, New York

Shauna Zorich, MD, MPH
Clinical Assistant Professor
Department of Epidemiology and
 Environmental Health
School of Public Health and Health
 Professions
University at Buffalo
Buffalo, New York

Michael LaMonte, PhD, MPH
Research Associate Professor
Department of Epidemiology and
 Environmental Health
School of Public Health and Health
 Professions
University at Buffalo
Buffalo, New York

Lina Mu, MD, PhD
Associate Professor
Department of Epidemiology and
 Environmental Health
School of Public Health and Health
 Professions
University at Buffalo
Buffalo, New York

▶ Chapter 2

Alicia L. Battle, PhD, MCHES
Assistant Professor
Department of Public Health
College of Education and
 Health Services
Benedictine University
Lisle, Illinois

Carolyn D. Rodgers, PhD, MHS, MCHES
Senior Lecturer
Addiction Studies Behavioral Health
Governors State University
University Park, Illinois

Shawnté Elbert, MA, MCHES, CHWC, TTS
Director
Office of Health and
 Wellness Promotion
Division of Student Affairs
Indiana University–Purdue
 University Indianapolis
Indianapolis, Indiana

▶ Chapter 3

Christopher S. Wichman, PhD
Assistant Professor
Department of Biostatistics
College of Public Health
University of Nebraska
 Medical Center
Omaha, Nebraska

Lynette M. Smith, PhD
Assistant Professor
Department of Biostatistics
College of Public Health
University of Nebraska Medical Center
Omaha, Nebraska

Paul A. Estabrooks, PhD
Professor and Howard M. Mauer
    Distinguished Chair
Department of Health Promotion
College of Public Health
University of Nebraska Medical Center
Omaha, Nebraska

▶ **Chapter 4**

Chantel D. Sloan, PhD
Assistant Professor
Department of Public Health
Brigham Young University
Provo, Utah

John D. Beard, PhD
Assistant Professor
Department of Public Health
Brigham Young University
Provo, Utah

▶ **Chapter 5**

Scott H. Frank, MD, MS
Associate Professor
Department of Population and
    Quantitative Health Sciences
Case Western Reserve University
    School of Medicine
Cleveland, Ohio

Matthew Kucmanic, MPH, MA
Public Health Specialist
Department of Population and
    Quantitative Health Sciences
Case Western Reserve University
    School of Medicine
Cleveland, Ohio

▶ **Chapter 6**

LeConté J. Dill, DrPH, MPH
Clinical Associate Professor and
    Director of Public Health Practice
College of Global Public Health
New York University
New York, New York

▶ **Chapter 7**

Nandi A. Marshall, DrPH, MPH, CHES
Assistant Professor
Jiann-Ping Hsu College of Public Health
Georgia Southern University
Statesboro, Georgia

Lynn D. Woodhouse, EdD, MPH
Professor Emeritus
East Stroudsburg University
East Stroudsburg, Pennsylvania

John S. Luque, PhD, MPH
Associate Professor
Institute of Public Health
Florida A&M University
Tallahassee, Florida

Gulzar H. Shah, PhD, MStat, MS
Department Chair and Associate
    Professor of Health Policy and
    Management
Jiann-Ping Hsu College of Public
    Health
Georgia Southern University
Statesboro, Georgia

Cassandra Arroyo, PhD, MS
Lead Statistical Analyst
Department of Research for Patient
    Care Services
Barnes-Jewish Hospital
St. Louis, Missouri

▶ Chapter 8

Elizabeth A. Baker, PhD, MPH, CPH
Assistant Professor
Department of Public Health
College of Health Sciences
Des Moines University
Des Moines, Iowa

▶ Chapter 9

Elizabeth Squires, MPH, MCHES
Clinical Professional Faculty
Department of Public Health
College of Education and Health
    Services
Benedictine University
Lisle, Illinois

David Milen, PhD
Department of Public Health
College of Education and Health
    Services
Benedictine University
Lisle, Illinois

▶ Chapter 10

Anthony J. Santella, DrPH, MCHES
Associate Professor
Department of Health Professions
Hofstra University
Hempstead, New York
Chair, Nassau–Suffolk Ryan
    White HIV Health Services
    Planning Council
Deer Park, New York

Georgette Beal, MHA
Senior Vice President, Planning and
    Grants Management
United Way of Long Island
Deer Park, New York

▶ Chapter 11

Spring Chenoa Cooper, PhD
Associate Professor
Department of Community Health
    and Social Sciences
CUNY Graduate School of Public
    Health and Health Policy
New York, New York

Claudia Wald, MSW
Research Coordinator
Department of Community Health
    and Social Sciences
CUNY Graduate School of Public
    Health and Health Policy
New York, New York

▶ Chapter 12

Jason M. Ackleson, PhD
Adjunct Faculty
Department of Diagnostic Medicine/
    Pathobiology
Kansas State University
Manhattan, Kansas

Sara E. Gragg, PhD
Assistant Professor
Department of Animal Sciences and
    Industry
Kansas State University
Manhattan, Kansas

Justin J. Kastner, PhD
Associate Professor
Department of Diagnostic
    Medicine/Pathobiology
Kansas State University
Manhattan, Kansas

Ellyn R. Mulcahy, PhD, MPH
Associate Professor
MPH Program Director
Department of Diagnostic Medicine/
    Pathobiology
Kansas State University
Manhattan, Kansas

Daniel A. Unruh, PhD
Research Assistant
Department of Animal Sciences and
    Industry
Kansas State University
Manhattan, Kansas

▶ **Chapter 13**

Cara L. Pennel, DrPH, MPH
Assistant Professor
Department of Preventive Medicine
    and Community Health
University of Texas Medical Branch
Galveston, Texas

John D. Prochaska, DrPH, MPH
Assistant Professor
Department of Preventive Medicine
    and Community Health
University of Texas Medical Branch
Galveston, Texas

Neilson Treble, LPC, ACPS
Family Engagement Specialist
21st Century ACE Cycle 9 Program
Texas City Independent School
    District
Texas City, Texas

Rob Ruffner, MPA
Executive Director
Galveston County Mutual Assistance
    Partnership
Texas City, Texas

Sharon Croisant, PhD, MS
Professor
Department of Preventive Medicine
    and Community Health
University of Texas Medical Branch
Galveston, Texas

▶ **Chapter 14**

Suzanne Carlberg-Racich, PhD, MSPH
Assistant Professor
Master of Public Health Program
DePaul University
Chicago, Illinois

▶ **Chapter 15**

Mark E. Gebhart, MD, FAAEM
Associate Professor
Department of Population and Public
    Health
Division of Health Systems and Policy
Wright State University Boonshoft
    School of Medicine
Dayton, Ohio

▶ **Chapter 16**

David M. Claborn, DrPH
Associate Professor
Master of Public Health Program
Missouri State University
Springfield, Missouri

▶ **Chapter 17**

Laura Erskine, PhD, MBA
Associate Adjunct Professor
MPH Program Director
Department of Health Policy and
    Management
UCLA Fielding School of Public
    Health
Los Angeles, California

▶ Chapter 18

Angela G. Clendenin, PhD, MA
Instructional Assistant Professor
Department of Epidemiology and
    Biostatistics
Texas A&M School of
    Public Health
College Station, Texas

▶ Chapter 19

Moya L. Alfonso, PhD, MSPH
Associate Professor
Department of Community Health
    Education and Behavior
Georgia Southern University
Statesboro, Georgia

Abraham Johnson, MPH
Former Student
Department of Community Health
    Education and Behavior
Georgia Southern University
Statesboro, Georgia

Jannapha Hubeny, BSPH
Former Student
Department of Community Health
    Education and Behavior
Georgia Southern University
Statesboro, Georgia

Maria Olivas, MPH
Doctoral Student
Department of Community Health
    Education and Behavior
Georgia Southern University
Statesboro, Georgia

▶ Chapter 20

Elizabeth A. Armstrong-Mensah, PhD, MIA
Clinical Assistant Professor
Department of Health Policy and
    Behavior Sciences
Georgia State University
Atlanta, Georgia

▶ Chapter 21

Anthony J. Santella, DrPH, MCHES
Associate Professor
Department of Health Professions
Hofstra University
Hempstead, New York

Gwen Cohen Brown, DDS, FAAOMP
Professor
Department of Dental Hygiene
New York City College of Technology
Brooklyn, New York

▶ Chapter 22

Kimberly Krytus, MSW, MPH, CPH
Director
MPH Initiatives
School of Public Health and Health
    Professions
University at Buffalo
Buffalo, New York

Gale Burstein, MD, MPH, FAAP
Commissioner of Health
Erie County Department of Health
Buffalo, New York

Dedication

*Dedicated to the public health professionals
who are tirelessly fighting for the rights of
those experiencing health inequities and
social injustices. Keep fighting the good fight!*

*Dedicated to my #1 supporter and partner,
Robbie. Everything will be perfect!*

Acknowledgments

I am thrilled to share the first edition of this public health case studies text. As a public health educator for the past 12 years, I have been frustrated with the dearth of public health practice-oriented case studies for Master of Public Health (MPH) students. In terms of the breadth and depth of topics and content, this text is the most comprehensive source of public health case studies available, and I am confident it will help prepare readers for a career in public health.

I could not have completed the book without the guidance and support of the Jones & Bartlett Learning staff, especially Michael Brown and Carter McAlister. I would also like to thank Thais Miller, Kelly Sylvester, Sophie Teague, and Susanne Walker for their assistance.

I also want to thank my family, friends, and Hofstra University colleagues, who have been a constant source of encouragement throughout this process.

Preface

The Council on Education in Public Health (CEPH) is recognized by the U.S. Department of Education as accrediting schools of public health and public health programs. To promote quality in public health education, CEPH, in consultation with the public health community, has established 22 foundational competencies that graduates of Master of Public Health (MPH) programs should have met by the end of their studies.

In 2016, new foundational MPH competencies were released, covering areas related to evidence-based approaches to public health, public health and healthcare systems, planning and management to promote health, policy in public health, leadership, communication, interprofessional practice, and systems thinking. These competencies are informed not only by the traditional public health core knowledge areas (biostatistics, epidemiology, social and behavioral sciences, health services administration, and environmental and occupational health) but also by cross-cutting and emerging public health areas.

Each chapter of the book focuses on one or more of the 22 CEPH MPH foundational competencies. Each chapter is also authored by a faculty member from a CEPH-accredited school of public health or public health program, often working with community partners, students, and practitioners. Each chapter consists of the following sections: background on a public health issue, the case study, case study summary points, application to CEPH competencies, discussion questions, and references.

I hope you find the book useful in the teaching and learning of the art and science of public health practice.

Evidence-Based Approaches to Public Health

CHAPTER 1

Epidemiologic Methods Applied in Various Settings of Public Health Practice

Ajay Anand Myneni, PhD, MBBS, MPH
Shauna Zorich, MD, MPH
Michael LaMonte, PhD, MPH
Lina Mu, MD, PhD

▶ Background

Epidemiology—with its primary goals of determining the causes and extent of disease, investigating the natural history of disease, evaluating preventive and therapeutic interventions, and informing public health policy and preventive medicine guidelines—contributes significantly to the mission of public health.[1,2] Epidemiologic methods are employed in a variety of study designs, and serve as powerful tools that find application in a broad range of public health settings. In this chapter, the utilization of epidemiologic methods to confront important health problems in a number of settings is described.

Setting 1: Public Health Surveillance

As an important tool to estimate the health status and behavior of a community, public health surveillance provides and interprets data to promote disease prevention and control.[3] The Behavioral Risk Factor Surveillance System (BRFSS), one such surveillance program, is an ongoing nationwide adult telephone survey conducted monthly, which collects data about behavior risk factors, chronic health conditions,

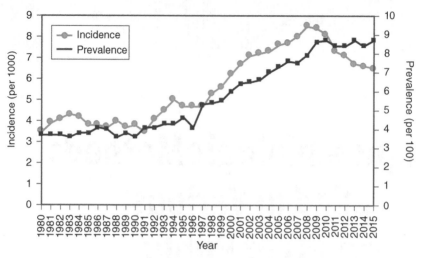

FIGURE 1-1 Trends in incidence and prevalence of diagnosed diabetes among U.S. adults, 1980–2015.

Data from: Centers for Disease Control and Prevention. (2018). *Diabetes report card 2017*. Retrieved from https://www.cdc.gov/diabetes/library/reports /congress.html

and use of preventive services.[4] Information collected in the BRFSS is applied in several important public health practices, one of which is the U.S. Diabetes Surveillance System (DSS). The DSS utilizes data from the BRFSS and the U.S. Census Bureau's Population Estimates Program to estimate and interpret annual prevalence and incidence of diagnosed diabetes at the county, state, and national levels.[5]

FIGURE 1-1 is reproduced from the Diabetes Report Card 2017,[6] which is a Centers for Disease Control and Prevention (CDC) publication based on findings from the DSS. This figure depicts the trends of incidence and prevalence of diabetes from 1980 to 2015. Both estimates show a steady increase over the years. However, there was a decreasing trend in incidence of diabetes from approximately 8.7 per 1000 population at risk in 2008 to 6.5 per 1000 in 2015. Estimates and trends such as these not only inform us about disease burden but also serve as an evaluation tool to assess the effectiveness of the existing intervention programs.

Setting 2: Public Health Research Studies

Prospective cohort studies are used to evaluate the *incidence* of a specified disease over time, and to determine whether there is a difference in disease incidence between study participants with and without an *exposure* of interest. An example of this type of study is the *Framingham Heart Study*, which is one of the most widely recognized and informative epidemiologic studies on the frequency and determinants of cardiovascular disease (CVD) conducted within the community setting.[7] Beginning in 1949, a general population sample of 5209 women and men, age 30–62 years, residing in the middle-class, relatively stable community of Framingham, Massachusetts, completed *baseline* assessments that included a blood collection, resting blood pressure and electrocardiogram, physical measures, and a detailed medical history. Every 2 years the examinations were repeated to update exposure information and to identify cases of CVD that had occurred since the previous visit.

The originally enrolled cohort represented 68% of the community members eligible, which requires epidemiologists to consider the extent to which this might introduce a *selection bias* in subsequent study results. *Follow-up* for incident cases of CVD over time, which is a critical component of the prospective cohort design, has been exceptional, with a greater than 95% completion rate. This high completion rate decreases the risk of a *loss to follow-up bias*.

One of the exposures of high interest in the Framingham Heart Study was resting blood pressure (BP), and its relationship with future development of CVD (e.g., heart attack, stroke). Adults who were without CVD at baseline had their BP measured and then were followed for an average of 11 years, during which 397 incident CVD cases were documented.[8] **FIGURE 1-2** shows the study findings. In both women and men, there is a *positive association* between baseline BP level and CVD incidence. The results shown are *adjusted* for age (a possible *confounder*) and are *sex-specific* (shown separately for women and men). Note that CVD incidence is higher in men than in women at each level of BP. The *relative risk* (incidence in exposed/incidence in nonexposed) can be used to compare CVD incidence between BP groups. In women, compared to those with the lowest BP (incidence = 1.9), the relative risks of incident CVD are 1.47 (3.8/1.9) and 2.32 (4.4/1.9) for those in the middle and highest categories, respectively. In other words, women in the middle and highest BP categories had 47% and 132% higher age-adjusted incidence of CVD as compared to women with the lowest BP.

Experimental studies, often called *randomized clinical trials* (or prevention trials), provide the strongest evidence of causality. In these studies, consenting and enrolled study participants are *assigned randomly*, or by *chance*, to be in the exposed (*intervention*) or nonexposed (*control*) group. Chance assignment balances all characteristics of participants between groups so that the only difference is

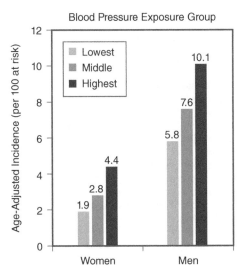

FIGURE 1-2 Cumulative incidence of CVD in adults followed for 11 years in the Framingham Heart Study.

Data from: Vasan, R. S., Larson, M. G., Leip, E. P., Evans, J. C., O'Donnell, C. J., Kannel, W. B., & Levy, D. (2001). Impact of high-normal blood pressure on the risk of cardiovascular disease. *New England Journal of Medicine, 345*(18), 1291–1297. doi:10.1056/NEJMoa003417

being exposed or not exposed. The study then proceeds much like the cohort study, with follow-up over time for incident disease and comparison of disease incidence between the intervention and control groups.

The *SPRINT trial* is a randomized prevention trial that evaluated whether lowering BP in adults with hypertension would decrease CVD incidence.[9] A total of 9361 adults, who had high BP at enrollment, were randomized to intensive drug therapy or usual treatment for hypertension and then followed for an average of 3 years for development of CVD. The incidence of CVD in the intervention group (intensive therapy) was 1.65 per 100 at risk per year, while the incidence of CVD in the control group (standard treatment) was 2.19 per 100 at risk per year. These results showed a clear benefit for CVD prevention in participants receiving intensive BP treatment as compared to those who received usual care. Because the intervention was assigned randomly, the assumption is that nothing other than exposure status differed between groups; thus the only factor that plausibly explains the difference in CVD incidence is exposure to the intervention. That is, the exposure caused the disease incidence to be lower in one group compared to the other. Importantly, results of observational studies, such as prospective cohorts, inform development and completion of randomized prevention trials to further evaluate a specific exposure–disease relationship in a manner that is most conclusive for cause and effect.

Setting 3: Outbreak Investigation

Outbreak investigation is one of the key applications of epidemiology in public health practice. "*Outbreak epidemiology* is the investigation of a disease cluster or epidemic with the goal of controlling or preventing further disease in a population."[10] Every outbreak investigation is handled slightly differently due to the varying nature of outbreaks. As a result, it is useful to utilize a systematic process when engaging in an outbreak investigation. The CDC has developed a list of steps (**FIGURE 1-3**) that investigators can apply when managing an outbreak.[3] Note that the

1. Prepare for field work
2. Establish the existence of an outbreak
3. Verify the diagnosis
4. Construct a working case definition
5. Find cases systematically and record information
6. Perform descriptive epidemiology
7. Develop hypotheses
8. Evaluate hypotheses epidemiologically
9. As necessary, reconsider, refine, and re-evaluate hypotheses
10. Compare and reconcile with laboratory and/or environmental studies
11. Implement control and prevention measures
12. Initiate or maintain surveillance
13. Communicate findings

FIGURE 1-3 Epidemiologic steps of an outbreak investigation.

steps may not be performed in this specific order and that multiple steps may be occurring simultaneously.

An *influenza outbreak at a military transit center in Kyrgyzstan* is reviewed here to illustrate a number of steps listed in Figure 1-3. The details of this outbreak have been published, and the features discussed here were derived from this publication.[11] The Transit Center at Manas, Kyrgyzstan, was the former gateway to Afghanistan; all troops moving into and out of Afghanistan passed through Manas. During the month of December 2013, only 7 individuals with influenza-like illness (ILI) had sought medical attention and 0 cases of influenza had been diagnosed. In early January 2014, medical personnel at Manas began to see a significant increase in the number of individuals seeking medical attention for ILI; on January 4, the first confirmed case of influenza was diagnosed. By mid-January, numerous individuals with ILI were seeking medical attention daily and more cases of influenza were being confirmed daily via laboratory analysis (**Step 3**). During the first 2 weeks of January, medical personnel identified 18 cases of laboratory-confirmed influenza, whereas 0 cases had been confirmed during the previous month of December. Medical personnel were aware that they were seeing a higher number of cases than expected, which helped to establish the existence of an outbreak (**Step 1**).

A *case definition* "is a standard set of criteria for deciding whether an individual should be classified as having the health condition of interest."[3] The following influenza-like illness case definition was established for this outbreak: oral temperature of 100.5°F or higher and cough or sore throat. Individuals considered to be cases of influenza were those with laboratory confirmation of influenza (**Step 4**). Laboratory confirmation was obtained by collecting respiratory specimens from ILI patients and testing the specimens for influenza A and B via polymerase chain reaction (PCR) (**Step 10**). Manas public health personnel maintained updated electronic line lists of all cases of ILI and confirmed influenza cases involved in the outbreak. Additional demographic and clinical information was collected for each case (**Step 5**). A total of 215 individuals met the case definition for ILI, and 85 individuals were determined to be laboratory-confirmed cases of influenza. All laboratory-confirmed influenza cases had been vaccinated (**Step 6**).

Public health personnel at Manas implemented numerous control measures to mitigate the outbreak. Isolation of influenza patients was the primary measure utilized; additional measures included strict hand washing, cough etiquette, education and awareness campaigns, and administration of antiviral medication for both the treatment and prevention of influenza (**Step 11**).

The last case of influenza occurred on February 14, 2014. The Transit Center at Manas continued to surveil for influenza-like illness cases until June 2014, when the Center was turned over to the Kyrgyz Republic (**Step 12**). Details of the outbreak as well as the outbreak response were communicated in various ways, including situation updates, influenza surveillance reports, and a published report in an academic military journal (**Step 13**).

Epidemiologic outbreak investigations like the one described here can help identify the etiology or cause of the outbreak, inform public health practitioners regarding proper control measures to mitigate the outbreak, and inform preventive measures that can be utilized to avert a similar outbreak in the future.

Summary Points

To sum up the review presented here, epidemiologic methods find significant application in the following areas:

1. The surveillance of important diseases to estimate their burden in the community and monitor trends over time, which helps in the planning and evaluation of intervention programs
2. Identifying risk factors of disease, and developing and evaluating therapeutic interventions
3. Investigating the etiology of outbreaks and informing control and preventive measures to confront and prevent similar outbreaks in the future

▶ Application of CEPH MPH Competencies

This case study addresses CEPH competencies 1, 2, 3, 4, and 5.

Competency 1: Apply Epidemiological Methods to the Breadth of Settings in Public Health Practice

In addition to the three previously mentioned areas, epidemiologic methods find their application in several other settings in public health practice: (1) identifying and prioritizing key health issues affecting the community; (2) developing and evaluating screening programs for deadly diseases such as cancer, enabling early treatment, and enhancing survival rates; and (3) evaluating the impact of public health interventions and policies.

Competency 2: Select Quantitative and Qualitative Data Collection Methods Appropriate for a Given Public Health Context

The BRFSS conducts telephone surveys to collect various quantitative data such as age, height, and weight.[12]

Competency 3: Analyze Quantitative and Qualitative Data Using Biostatistics, Informatics, Computer-Based Programming, and Software, as Appropriate; Competency 4: Interpret Results of Data Analysis for Public Health Research, Policy, and Practice

As described in the three previously mentioned settings, data collected using various study designs are analyzed using appropriate statistical methods and analytical software to derive useful study estimates such as incidence, prevalence, and relative risks. Careful and accurate interpretation of these estimates contributes to public health research and facilitates development of guidelines for public health policy and practice.

Competency 5: Design a Population-Based Policy, Program, Project, or Intervention

The application of epidemiologic evidence from observational studies and randomized prevention trials to clinical and public health practice is best appreciated through the development and implementation of guidelines aimed at improving population health. An example is the recently published blood pressure guidelines in the United States.[13] Evidence from several published studies, utilizing a variety of study designs, including the two studies referenced previously, were evaluated by an expert panel. This panel then wrote practice guidelines to aid healthcare providers in managing the blood pressure of their patients, and to aid public health practitioners in developing community-level education and screening programs.

Discussion Questions

1. How can you evaluate the effectiveness of an intervention program designed to reduce disease burden in the community using public health surveillance?
2. How do prospective cohort studies and randomized controlled trials differ in their application in public health practice?
3. Discuss the principal findings from the Framingham Heart Study and the *SPRINT trial* on the relationship between blood pressure and cardiovascular disease.
4. When engaging in an epidemiologic outbreak investigation, why is it important to uncover the etiology or cause of the outbreak?
5. If you were asked to identify the three most important steps of an outbreak investigation, which would you identify and why?

References

1. Gordis, L. (2014). *Epidemiology* (5th ed.). Philadelphia, PA: Elsevier Saunders.
2. Institute of Medicine. (1988). *The future of public health*. Washington, DC: National Academies Press.
3. Centers for Disease Control and Prevention. (2012). *Principles of epidemiology in public health practice: An introduction to applied epidemiology and biostatistics* Retrieved from https://www.cdc.gov/ophss/csels/dsepd/ss1978/ss1978.pdf
4. Centers for Disease Control and Prevention. (2018, April 25). Behavioral Risk Factor Surveillance System. Retrieved from https://www.cdc.gov/brfss/
5. Centers for Disease Prevention and Control. (2018). United States Diabetes Surveillance System: Data and statistics. Retrieved from https://www.cdc.gov/diabetes/data/index.html
6. Centers for Disease Control and Prevention. (2018). *Diabetes report card 2017*. Retrieved from https://www.cdc.gov/diabetes/library/reports/congress.html
7. LaMonte, M. J. (2008). Epidemiology of cardiovascular disease. In J. L. Durstine, G. Moore, M. J. LaMonte, & B. A. Franklin (Eds.), *Pollock's textbook of cardiovascular disease and rehabilitation* (pp. 9–22). Champaign, IL: Human Kinetics.
8. Vasan, R. S., Larson, M. G., Leip, E. P., Evans, J. C., O'Donnell, C. J., Kannel, W. B., & Levy, D. (2001). Impact of high-normal blood pressure on the risk of cardiovascular disease. *New England Journal of Medicine, 345*(18), 1291–1297. doi:10.1056/NEJMoa003417
9. SPRINT Research Group. (2015). A randomized trial of intensive versus standard blood-pressure control. *New England Journal of Medicine, 373*(22), 2103–2116. doi:10.1056/NEJMoa1511939

10. Dwyer, D. M., Groves, C., & Blythe, D. (2014). Outbreak epidemiology. In K. E. Nelson & C. M. Williams (Eds.), *Infectious disease epidemiology theory and practice* (pp. 105–129). Burlington, MA: Jones & Bartlett Learning.

11. Parms, T. A., Zorich, S. C., & Kramer, K. P. (2015). Influenza A (H3N2) outbreak at transit center at Manas, Kyrgyzstan, 2014. *Medical Surveillance Monthly Report, 22*(1).

12. Centers for Disease Control and Prevention. (2018, April 30). National Health and Nutrition Examination Survey. Retrieved from https://www.cdc.gov/nchs/nhanes/index.htm

13. Whelton, P. K., Carey, R. M., Aronow, W. S., Casey, D. E., Collins, K. J., Dennison Himmelfarb, C., . . . Wright, J. T. (2018). 2017 ACC/AHA/AAPA/ABC/ACPM/AGS/APhA/ASH /ASPC/NMA/PCNA guideline for the prevention, detection, evaluation, and management of high blood pressure in adults. *A Report of the American College of Cardiology/American Heart Association Task Force on Clinical Practice Guidelines, 71*(19), e127–e248. doi:10.1016/j .jacc.2017.11.00

CHAPTER 2

Mixed Methods for Evaluating Alcohol Norms, Access, and Behaviors Among Youth in Chicago Heights, Illinois

Alicia L. Battle, PhD, MCHES
Carolyn D. Rodgers, PhD, MHS, MCHES
Shawnté Elbert, MA, MCHES, CHWC, TTS

▶ Background

Located 24 miles directly south of the Chicago Loop, Chicago Heights has a rich history with its industrial beginnings and its pride in being the "Crossroads of the Nations," as the site of the intersection of the first two transcontinental highways in the United States.[1] The Lincoln and Dixie Highways, the railroads, and the many industries in the area created a booming community of immigrant workers—Polish, Italian, Slovak, Irish, Lithuanian, Mexican, and African American.[1,2] According to the U.S. Census Bureau, in 2016, the residents of Chicago Heights self-identified as Black (41.7%), Hispanic (32.6%), and White (23.2%); some residents self-identified as two or more races (1.49%) and as "other" (0.75%).[3,4] In 2016, the median age of the residents in Chicago Heights was 34 years of age, with nearly 27% being younger than age 18.[3,4] The median household income of Chicago Heights was $40,611—less than the national, state, and county averages.[3,4] The average income in Chicago Heights for males was 1.13 times higher than the average income of females, with an income inequality of 0.426—lower than the national average.[3,4] Females accounted for a predominant portion of the student population in Chicago Heights, with 389 male students and 804 female students in the population (52% females and 48% males).[3,4]

Alcohol is the most widely abused drug among adolescents in the United States.[5] Motor vehicle crashes involving alcohol consumption are the most significant mortality risk issue facing youth age 12–20 years.[6] Alcohol consumption accounts for more than 4300 deaths among U.S. youth annually.[7,8] Individuals between the ages of 12 and 20 are responsible for approximately 11% of all the alcohol consumed in the country—with more than 90% of this amount consumed in the form of binge drinking. Alcohol consumption during adolescence and early adolescence increases the odds of future physical and behavioral health problems.[9,10] Abuse of other drugs, increased risk for suicide and homicide, and social problems are critical trends to focus on in association with youth alcohol use. The likelihood of developing alcohol dependence or abuse later in life is 6 times greater among those who began drinking before the age of 15 years as compared to those who started drinking at the legal age of 21 years or later.[10] There is also a greater risk of abuse and dependence of other substances in adulthood—such as marijuana, inhalants, and cocaine and other psychostimulants—among individuals who began substance use in adolescence or early adolescence.[9]

The most widespread consumption pattern for the 12- to 20-year-old age group is binge drinking. Binge drinking, as defined by Substance Abuse and Mental Health Services Administration (SAMHSA), is the consumption of five or more alcoholic beverages in one sitting within the past 30 days. Research indicates that adolescents who drink are more likely to experience disruptions of normal growth and sexual development, higher risk of suicide, and changes in brain development. It was in part for these reasons that, in 2007, the Surgeon General's Call to Action to Prevent and Reduce Underage Drinking encouraged coordination and partnerships among government, the private sector, and individuals to reduce underage alcohol consumption.[11] This initiative followed the release of a report (*Reducing Underage Drinking: A Collective Responsibility*) in 2003 by the National Research Council and Institute of Medicine, wherein the alcohol industry, alcohol retailers, community-based organizations, and parents were exhorted to coordinate their efforts directed toward reductions in youth alcohol use.[5]

▶ Case Study

The Chicago Heights South Suburban Family Wellness Alliance (SSFWA) was built upon the success of the Family Wellness Program (FWP), which began in 1991. The FWP aimed to complement and enhance communities' existing Head Start programs, targeting families in seven suburban communities by collaborating with their local Head Start centers. The SSFWA's mission is to holistically address health disparities among City of Chicago Heights residents; support the development of healthy individuals and families in the community through advocacy, education, policy, systems, and environmental change; and engage community stakeholders to collaboratively work toward an enhanced caring and inclusive climate for all citizens. The SSFWA was formally established in July 2009 as a substance use prevention and behavioral and public health promotion coalition, composed of key community stakeholders with the vision of significantly reducing underage drinking and illegal drug use by youth. The primary target populations for SSFWA's work are youth and their families in Chicago Heights. The SSFWA utilizes the U.S. Department of Health and Human Services, SAMHSA, and Center for Substance Abuse Prevention (CSAP) Strategic Prevention Framework, with the intention of identifying key issues and effecting positive community change through assessment, capacity building, planning, evidence-based strategy implementation, and evaluation, with an emphasis on alcohol and other drug prevention but also including general health promotion.

In September 2013, SSFWA was awarded a SAMHSA CSAP Drug Free Communities (DFC) grant. The project period for the award was September 30, 2013, through September 29, 2018. The award of $125,000.00 per year for 5 years was to be used to (1) establish and strengthen collaboration among communities, public and private nonprofit agencies, and federal, state, local, and tribal governments and (2) support prevention programs and services designed to reduce substance use among youth. In accepting the project award, SSFWA was required to comply with DFC evaluation provisions. These included data collected every 2 years on use of alcohol, tobacco, marijuana, and prescription drugs for three grades (6–12) with a combination of odd or even years capturing two high school grades. The data collected also encompassed the following:

- Past 30-day use
- Perception of risk or harm
- Perception of parental disapproval of use
- Perception of peer disapproval of use

Using both quantitative and qualitative methods, a group of Governors State University student volunteers conducted a community assessment of Chicago Heights. The quantitative methods employed included administration of surveys and the examination of secondary data. The qualitative methods employed included observation, focus groups, and individual interviews. The student volunteers spent 12 weeks in the field collecting data to complete the following worksheets and tools: (1) Promotion and Advertisement Worksheets; (2) Retail Availability/Bar Assessment Tool, (3) Enforcement (Alcohol and Marijuana Assessment Tools), (4) Community Alcohol Access Assessment Tool; and (5) Community Norms Worksheet

Data were collected by administering surveys, facilitation of both individual and focus group interviews, and field observation. Students also used data from the Illinois Youth Survey administered in 2014. There were two key findings:

- The results showed an enormous number of alcohol outlets (*especially liquor stores*) in the community. There are currently 146 active liquor licenses, but this number does not include the unknown number of businesses supplying alcohol that operate without a license.
- The results indicated that the physical environment lends itself to the creation of unsafe social normative behaviors.

Given these two key findings, the following recommendations were provided to serve as a starting point for the development of programs and were intended to speak to the access that youth in Chicago Heights have to alcohol. Additionally, the recommendations were intended to guide the development of programs and services targeted at youth that address alcohol norms and behaviors.

Summary Points

1. Chicago Heights South Suburban Family Wellness Alliance (SSFWA) was established in 2009 to address health disparities. SSFWA is a substance use prevention and behavioral and public health promotion coalition, composed of key community stakeholders with the vision of significantly reducing underage drinking and illegal drug use by youth.

2. A 5-year grant of $125,000 per year for 5 years was awarded to SSFWA to (1) establish and strengthen collaboration and (2) support the creation and sustainment of prevention programs and services that will reduce substance use among youth.

3. Public health students participated in both qualitative and quantitative methods over 12 weeks, to gather data on the use and perceptions of substance abuse within the community.

4. There is an extremely high saturation of alcohol stores and liquor licenses within the Chicago Heights community. This increases environmental factors that create unhealthy behaviors and perceptions on substance abuse.

5. Key recommendations made based on the study results included establishing an alcohol prevention program in the schools; increasing promotion of safe drinking in Chicago Heights at public events; reexamining zoning ordinances with regard to proximity to schools and daycare facilities; establishing, enacting, and enforcing strict loitering policies for all alcohol outlets; more strictly enforcing alcohol laws; and obtaining funding for the built environment (e.g., restoring sidewalks, improving parks, getting rid of abandoned buildings and blighted homes).

▶ Application of CEPH MPH Competencies

Public health research boasts many studies that make use of both quantitative and qualitative methods. While quantitative and qualitative methods work to examine two completely different perspectives of an event (e.g., program, policy, service, intervention), these methods can be combined for complementary purposes. The case study here utilized both methods. The methods were used as a preliminary qualitative inquiry to make meaning of existing quantitative data or as a follow-up method to better understand the data gathered. This case study addresses CEPH competencies 2 and 11.

Competency 2: Select Quantitative and Qualitative Data Collection Methods Appropriate for a Given Public Health Context

Student volunteers were responsible for demonstrating several skills in conducting the community assessment within the Chicago Heights community. First, students needed to demonstrate an understanding of the logic model. In this instance, student volunteers were to use the logic model to understand, plan, develop, and evaluate prevention-based programs and community norms regarding alcohol use. Second, student volunteers demonstrated and used quantitative and qualitative methods to develop a logic model to create a conceptual design of an ideal program based on conducting a literature review of empirical data for best practices. Third, student volunteers facilitated focus groups, conducted individual interviews, and attended community meetings to observe and document strategies developed and approved by key stakeholders, community members, SSFWA coalition members, and the lead faculty evaluator. Additionally, student volunteers developed strategies from qualitative and quantitative results of community assessments from surveys, focus groups, and literature reviews to determine the best theoretical approach and practices for alcohol prevention-based program development. Afterward, student volunteers under the supervision of the faculty leader developed a conceptual design to implement and evaluate programs within the Chicago Heights community.

Competency 11: Select Methods to Evaluate Public Health Programs

Using the public health model students, volunteers were expected to demonstrate knowledge of the evaluation process and the four types of evaluations: formative, process, impact and outcome, and a summative report. Student volunteers were given the Centers for Disease Control and Prevention's (CDC's) recommended framework for evaluation to make sure effective evaluation was completed. The first two steps in this framework are engaging stakeholders and describing the program. Student volunteers engaged stakeholders from Chicago Heights to ensure community involvement, partnership, and utility of services. Utility of services was established by student volunteers surveying community members by conducting a formative evaluation. The formative evaluation included a systematic literature review of evidence-based programs and services appropriate for a population similar to the demographics of Chicago Heights, so as to develop program goals, objectives, and expected outcomes. Student volunteers under the supervision of the lead faculty evaluator conducted a SWOT (strengths, weaknesses, opportunities, threats) analysis using best practices and approaches to determine the feasibility, propriety, and accuracy of the programs.

Once feasibility was established and the programs were approved and finalized, phase 2 of the evaluation began. This phase included student volunteers under the supervision of the lead faculty focusing the evaluation design on program objectives. Developing and focusing the evaluation design required the inclusion of a process evaluation, which encompassed continuous monitoring and tracking of the number of people participating during each program session, activity, and service.

The third phase included an outcome evaluation of short- and long-term program objectives. Students under the supervision of the lead faculty evaluator assessed changes in behaviors and program objectives.

The final phase of the evaluation included an impact evaluation and confirmation of the accuracy of the results. Student volunteers collected impact data via a survey of knowledge, attitudes, and behavioral norms regarding alcohol use in the community. Student volunteers, under the supervision of the lead faculty evaluator, documented the program results and participated in recording all findings in a summative report that was later delivered and distributed to stakeholders, SSFWA members, and the grant-sponsoring agency for reporting purposes.

Discussion Questions

1. Describe the qualitative methods employed by the student volunteers. How do these methods capture the DFC evaluation's required data? List other qualitative research methods that the student volunteers may have used to glean the same information.

2. Describe the quantitative methods employed by the student volunteers. How do these methods capture the DFC evaluation's required data? Share the limitations of each method used and suggest at least two ways to mitigate these limitations.

3. Given the two key findings in the case, are the recommendations reasonable? Why or why not? Provide support for your position.

References

1. Craig, K. (2011). *History and related facts of the City of Chicago Heights*. Chicago Heights Public Library. Retrieved from https://static1.squarespace.com/static/531d92b8e4b025f658487979/t/5320d448e4b07843983669dc/1394660424279/HistoryofCHinbrief2.pdf

2. Chicago Heights. (2017). *Chicago gang history*. Retrieved from https://chicagoganghistory.com/suburb/chicago-heights/

3. U.S. Census Bureau. (2016). American Community Survey 5-year estimates [Data file]. *Census Reporter: Chicago Heights, IL*. Retrieved from https://censusreporter.org/profiles/16000US1714026-chicago-heights-il/

4. Chicago Heights, IL. (2016). *DataUSA*. Retrieved from https://datausa.io/profile/geo/chicago-heights-il/#demographics

5. National Institute on Alcohol Abuse and Alcoholism. (2007). *Underage drinking: Highlights from The Surgeon General's call to action to prevent and reduce underage drinking*. Rockville, MD: U.S. Department of Health and Human Services, National Institutes of Health, National Institute on Alcohol Abuse and Alcoholism.

6. Harding, F. M., Hingson, R. W., Klitzner, M., Mosher, J. F., Brown, J., Vincent, R. M., & Dahl, E. (2016). Underage drinking: A review of trends and prevention strategies. *American Journal of Preventive Medicine, 51*(42), 148–157.

7. Institute of Medicine. (2003). *Reducing underage drinking: A collective responsibility*. Washington, DC: National Academy of Sciences.

8. Sacks, J. J., Gonzales, K. R., Bouchery, E. E., Tomedi, L. E., & Brewer, R. D. (2015). 2010 national and state costs of excessive alcohol consumption. *American Journal of Preventive Medicine, 49*(5), e73–e79. doi:10.1016/j.amepre.2015.05.031

9. Substance Abuse and Mental Health Services Administration. (2016). *Risk and protective factors and estimates of substance use initiation: Results from the 2015 national survey on drug use and health*. Retrieved from https://www.samhsa.gov/data/report/risk-and-protective-factors-and-estimates-substance-use-initiation-results-2015-national

10. Substance Abuse and Mental Health Services Administration. (2017). *Report to Congress on the prevention and reduction of underage drinking*. Rockville, MD: U.S. Department of Health and Human Services.

11. Office of the Surgeon General, National Institute on Alcohol Abuse and Alcoholism, & Substance Abuse and Mental Health Services Administration. (2007). *The Surgeon General's call to action to prevent and reduce underage drinking: NCBI bookshelf*. Retrieved from http://www.ncbi.nlm.nih.gov/books/NBK44360

CHAPTER 3

Overweight Children: Analysis of Three Interventions in Reducing BMI *z*-Scores

Christopher S. Wichman, PhD
Lynette M. Smith, PhD
Paul A. Estabrooks, PhD

▶ Background

Childhood obesity has well-documented relationships with reduced physical, social, and psychological health and predisposes children to experiencing chronic disease as adults.[1] An obese child is more likely to be obese as an adult and to suffer from metabolic syndrome.[2] Metabolic syndrome in adolescents is defined as a collection of risk factors for type 2 diabetes and cardiovascular disease.[3] Aside from metabolic syndrome, obesity in adulthood has been associated with increased risks of multiple types of cancer, cognitive dysfunction, sleep apnea, and non-alcoholic fatty liver disease.[4]

Childhood obesity in the United States has been at epidemic levels since at least 1985.[5] An analysis of the 2013–2014 National Health and Nutrition Examination Survey (NHANES) completed in 2016 estimated that 17.2% and 16.2% of people age 2–19 years in the United States are classified as obese and overweight by the Centers for Disease Control and Prevention (CDC) definitions, respectively.[6] The epidemic of childhood obesity is not restricted to the United States alone; this is a worldwide issue. In fact, the World Health Organization (WHO) has identified childhood obesity as "one of the most serious public health challenges of the 21st century"; in 105 out of 194 reporting countries, the prevalence of obesity is 20% or higher.[7]

In 2014, it was estimated that obesity accounts for between 2% and 7% of healthcare spending in developed economies or roughly 2.8% of global gross domestic product (GDP).[8] The U.S. National Institutes of Health (NIH) spent $3.534 billion on obesity research alone between FY2013 and FY2016 and expect to spend an additional $1.777 billion on obesity research in FY2017 and FY2018.[9] The level of funding, the economic impact, and the increased risk of morbidities indicate that childhood obesity remains an important focus area for NIH, and for clinical, behavioral, and public health researchers.

▶ Case Study

Between May 2004 and February 2007, a team of researchers partnered with Kaiser Permanente Colorado to explore the viability and relative efficacy of an additive intervention in curbing overweight and obesity in adolescents.[10] To address this goal, the research team designed and implemented a longitudinal, three-group, randomized controlled trial. A unique feature of the study was that the unit of randomization was the parent–child dyad, such that the intervention was directly "applied" to the parent and the observations were taken on the child.[11] The primary outcome measure was the child's body mass index (BMI) z-score, which is a reflection of weight status. Secondary measures included self-report of physical activity and sedentary behavior (PA/SB); fruit, vegetable, and sugared-drink consumption; and eating disorder symptoms.

Each of the three levels of the intervention were scalable, additive, and designed for external validity and generalizability within a healthcare context. Group 1 received the Family Connections workbook (FC-WB); group 2 received FC-WB plus two FC-small group (FC-SG) sessions; and group 3 received FC-WB and FC-SG plus 10 interactive voice response (IVR) phone calls. The FC-WB is a 61-page workbook divided into two parts. Part 1 includes activities that encourage parents to examine the home environment and its influence on eating and physical activity, the causes of obesity, the short- and long-term impacts of obesity, and ways to promote healthy habits at home. Part 2 focuses on implementing changes in the home environment and parenting skills to promote healthy choices and activities in the home. The workbook provides activities that can be completed over a 5-day period.

FC-SG added two clinic-based, dietician-led small-group sessions, with a 1-week interval between sessions. Group sizes ranged from 10 to 15 parents. The first session focused on parenting skills and education about physical activity and healthy eating. The second session focused on making structural changes in the home to support a healthier lifestyle.

The IVR intervention utilized telephone contacts spaced out over 20 weeks after completion of the second FC-small group. IVR contact frequency was modulated: weekly for weeks 1 through 4; every other week from week 6 to 12; and finally, at weeks 16 and 20. The last IVR contact focused on relapse prevention. The IVR contacts sought to reinforce the concepts and knowledge gained from the FC-WB and FC-SG sessions, such as nutrition, healthy habits, physical activity, goal setting, and weight management. A secondary purpose was to determine whether the number of IVR contacts had any effect on outcomes. To address this question, three post-hoc groups were formed: FC-WB and FC-SG combined, and FC-IVR divided into two subgroups (those completing five or fewer IVR contacts and those completing six or more IVR contacts). Outcomes were then compared between these groups.

An a priori sample-size analysis indicated that 64 dyads per group were needed to detect a small effect between groups, assuming a significance level of 0.05 with a power of 0.80. Because interest was primarily focused on the difference between FC-SG and FC-IVR, more dyads were randomized to these two groups than to FC-WB, in a ratio of 1.7 to 1. To be included, a family needed a child between 8 and 12 years of age with a BMI greater than or equal to the 85th percentile. Families that expected to move out of the geographic area prior to the end of the study or whose physician asked they not be contacted were excluded from consideration. Over the course of the study, 1487 families were identified as potential participants, of which 656 were assessed. Ultimately, 220 were randomized to one of the three groups: 50 to FC-WB; 85 to FC-SG; and 85 to FC-IVR.

Each of the primary and secondary outcomes was measured at three time points: baseline (BL), 6 months, and 12 months. The BMI z-score is the preferred outcome measure for evaluating an intervention's impact in children and adolescents as compared to percentile or weight gain/loss because it is continuous and simultaneously takes into account changes in height and weight due to the natural progression of the maturity of subjects. Three questionnaires were used to collect self-report measures on behavior, food consumption, and eating disorders. Demographic variables of age, gender, and race/ethnicity were collected at baseline. Following randomization, groups were compared across outcome and demographic variables, to check for any indication of a priori differences that could influence the results.

Analyses for both the primary and secondary purposes were completed using the intent-to-treat principle. "Intent to treat" indicates that any subject who was randomized to a treatment group will be analyzed as a member of that group regardless of compliance with the assigned regimen. Primary and secondary outcomes were analyzed using generalized linear mixed models due to their ability to handle both normal and non-normal outcome variables and the longitudinal nature of the study.

Analysis 1 for BMI z-scores showed that all three groups exhibited a decrease over time. Detectable decreases in BMI z-score were observed between baseline and 12 months for FC-WB; between baseline and 6 months for FC-SG, but not sustained at 12 months; and between baseline and 6 and 12 months for FC-IVR. The difference between intervention groups was not detectable. Aside from FC-IVR showing a detectable increase in the number of days of moderate physical activity (MPA), none of the secondary outcomes showed any detectable changes across time or between groups.

In analysis 2, the FC-IVR group was broken out into 20 dyads having five or fewer phone contacts and 38 dyads having six or more phone contacts. The FC-IVR dyads completing six or more phone contacts demonstrated a decrease in BMI z-score from baseline to 6 and 12 months, while those completing five or fewer phone contacts did not. The FC-IVR six or more contacts group also demonstrated larger decreases than the FC-WB and FC-SG groups. Similar to analysis 1, the only secondary outcome showing any change was MPA. Specifically, the FC-IVR six or more contacts group demonstrated an increase in MPA from baseline to 6 and 12 months.

The research team ultimately concluded "automated telephone counseling can support parents of overweight children to reduce the extent to which their children are overweight."

Summary Points

1. Longitudinal randomized controlled trial: The goal was to establish the efficacy of a scalable, additive intervention to address the childhood overweight and obesity epidemic.
2. Nontraditional design: The experimental unit was the parent–child dyad, with the intervention applied directly to the parent and observation done on the child.
3. Preplanned secondary analyses: Alternative hypotheses were generated a priori as a backup plan in the event that the primary hypotheses could not be confirmed.
4. The study setting was a private health system with multiple and varied providers to improve external validity.

▶ Application of CEPH MPH Competencies

This case study addresses CEPH competencies 2, 3, and 4.

Competency 2: Select Quantitative and Qualitative Data Collection Methods Appropriate for a Given Public Health Context

The goal of this study was to demonstrate the relative efficacy of a scalable, additive intervention to address the childhood overweight and obese epidemic. The researchers chose BMI z-score as the primary outcome and secondary outcomes related to physical activity, eating habits, and eating disorders. BMI z-scores convert the traditional calculated BMI based on a subject's height and weight into normalized scores based on the subject's gender and age. To minimize biases due to measurement and calculation error, height and weight were measured in the clinic at each visit and centrally converted into BMI z-score using an algorithm developed by the CDC. The use of BMI and the z-score in particular is important for adolescents, given that they are still in the growth phase of life. The secondary outcomes were chosen because they are readily accepted as indicators for overweight and obesity. Physical activity measures were collected at each time point as the number of days of moderate and vigorous activity per week; sedentary behavior was quantified as the number of hours of being sedentary plus screen time per day. Sugared-drink, vegetable, and fruit consumption was collected using frequency and amount self-reports. The amount consumed was converted to servings using the U.S. Department of Agriculture nutrient database. All behavioral assessments used existing self-reported measures that could be used to compare to regional prevalence. Data were entered and stored in wide format (in which each row represented a single child) in a simple spreadsheet application.

Qualitative data were gathered using research field notes throughout the recruitment process and at each assessment point. Those data were reduced to themes and used for quality improvement—specific to methods to engage families in weight management interventions. One unique qualitative finding was that parents were more likely to participate when they received a letter from their physician as compared to being referred to the program during a clinical visit. Parents indicated that they felt more motivated to join the study when the pediatrician was concerned enough to reach out to them outside of the typical visit. In relation to the FC-IVR intervention, parents also felt more positively about the telephone system and recommended that it become part of typical pediatrics practice.

Competency 3: Analyze Quantitative and Qualitative Data Using Biostatistics, Informatics, Computer-Based Programming, and Software, as Appropriate

All analyses were conducted using SAS version 9.1. Generalized linear mixed models (GLMM) were used to analyze the effect of treatment group and time. Changes in BMI z-score and the square root of dietary outcomes over time and differences between groups were analyzed via linear mixed models (LMM). LMMs are a subclass of the GLMM; LMMs model the expected value of the outcome directly and assume that both error and any random effects are distributed normally with a mean of zero and fixed, but separate, variance components for each random effect. In this study, the subject was treated as a random effect. When the subject is treated as random, the within-subjects variability is the covariance between adjacent observations on the same subject. The square root transformation of dietary outcomes was needed to meet the LMM assumption of constant error variance.

The researchers chose to model the logit physical activity rate (days per week / hours per day) across time and between groups using a binomial GLMM. When rates are appropriately converted into proportions (proportion of week spent in physical activity / proportion of day spent sedentary), the observation is converted from a count per fixed time interval into a dimensionless value restricted between 0 and 1. As with the LMM, the GLMM takes into account the correlation of multiple measures on the same subject by treating the individual as a random block (also known as random intercept). The variance component of the random intercept thus becomes the covariance between observations on the same individual and is assumed to be the same for all individuals.

Qualitative information was gathered as part of the intervention delivery for FC-IVR. Parents provided feedback relative to goal progress that aligned with either (1) completely reaching previous goals, (2) making progress but not quite reaching goals, or (3) not making progress. Based on the response, an automated, branching-logic algorithm determined the content of the support message—with goal that achieving and progressing parents would receive reinforcing messages and reminders and that not progressing parents would receive messages intended to improve parental self-efficacy to make home environmental changes. Further, the FC-IVR was an adaptation of an evidence-based intervention and used previous program participant feedback and success to develop population-specific messaging that would resonate with future program participants. The phrases and short statements were then presented to focus groups, who were asked to comment on the impact and understandability of the content. The results of the focus group were used to determine the most impactful and readily understandable phrasing for the largest number of people.

Competency 4: Interpret Results of Data Analysis for Public Health Research, Policy, or Practice

The authors noted that when compared to baseline, all levels of the intervention showed modest decreases in BMI z-score during at least one of the follow time points. In their discussion, they readily admit that future research is needed to determine the frequency and duration of the FC-IVR contacts to achieve the optimal decrease in and maintain the loss in BMI z-score. With regard to practice, this study demonstrated that academic researchers partnered with non-research-based practices and health systems can work together in developing programs to address childhood overweight and obesity. The FC-IVR intervention was later adapted to a six-call program that was taken to scale within the healthcare system after the research was completed (accessible at innovations.ahrq.gov).

Discussion Questions

1. To be scalable, an intervention must be easy to extend across multiple entities with little to no training. How does the intervention used in this study rate as being scalable?
2. Do the additive levels of this intervention translate to any state within the United States? What about to any country across the globe?
3. In their discussion, the authors identify the fact that parents were not randomized to the number of IVR contacts, making it impossible to determine if parent motivation or number of IVR contacts explains the decrease in BMI z-score between those with six or more phone contacts versus five or fewer phone contacts. Why is this an appropriate conclusion?
4. How does this randomized controlled trial help address the childhood overweight and obesity epidemic?
5. The study does not include a true control group (a group not receiving an intervention). Would it have been ethical to include a control group? Why or why not?

References

1. Deckelbaum, R. J., & Williams, C. L. (2001). Childhood obesity: The health issue. *Obesity Research, 9,* 239S–243S.
2. Biro, F. M., & Wien, M. (2010). Childhood obesity and adult morbidities. *American Journal of Clinical Nutrition, 91*(5), 1499S–1505S.
3. International Diabetes Federation. (2006). The IDF consensus worldwide definition of the metabolic syndrome. Retrieved from https://www.idf.org/e-library/consensus-statements /60-idfconsensus-worldwide-definitionof-the-metabolic-syndrome.html
4. Mitchell, N., Catenacci, V., Wyatt, H. R., & Hill, J. O. (2011). Obesity: Overview of an epidemic. *Psychiatric Clinics of North America, 34*(4), 717–732. doi:10.1016/j.psc.2011.08.005
5. Dietz, W. H., Gortmaker, S. L., Sobol, A. M., Wehler, C. A., & Grand, R. J. (1985). Trends in the prevalence of childhood obesity in the United States. *Pediatric Research, 19,* 198A.

6. Fryar, C. D., Carroll, M. D., & Ogden, C. L. (2016). Prevalence of overweight and obesity among children and adolescents aged 2-19 years: United States, 1963–1965 through 2013–2014. Retrieved from https://www.cdc.gov/nchs/data/hestat/obesity_child_13_14/obesity _child_13_14.pdf

7. World Health Organization, Global Strategy on Diet, Physical Activity and Health. (2016). Childhood overweight and obesity. Retrieved from http://www.who.int/dietphysicalactivity /childhood/en/

8. McKinsey Global Institute. (2014, November). *Overcoming obesity: An initial economic analysis.* Retrieved from https://www.mckinsey.com/~/media/McKinsey/Business%20 Functions/Economic%20Studies%20TEMP/Our%20Insights/How%20the%20world %20could%20better%20fight%20obesity/MGI_Overcoming_obesity_Full_report.ashx

9. National Institutes of Health. (2017). Estimates of funding for various research, condition, and disease categories (RCDC). Retrieved from https://report.nih.gov/categorical_spending.aspx

10. Estabrooks, P. A., Shoup, J. A., Gattshall, M., Dandamudi, P., Shetterly, S., & Xu, S. (2009). Automated telephone counseling for parents of overweight children: A randomized controlled trial. *American Journal of Preventive Medicine, 36*(1), 35–42.

11. Golan, M., Fainaru, M., & Weizman, A. (1998). Role of behaviour modification in the treatment of childhood obesity with parents as the exclusive agents of change. *International Journal of Obesity, 22*, 1217–1222.

CHAPTER 4

Designing Policy to Reduce Particulate Matter Air Concentrations in Cache County, Utah

Chantel D. Sloan, PhD
John D. Beard, PhD

▶ Background

Exposure to air pollution can result in adverse health effects.[1] Small particulates in the air increase inflammation in the cardiovascular and respiratory systems and aggravate existing health conditions.[2] This is especially true for children, the elderly, and individuals with pulmonary or cardiovascular conditions.[3,4]

The effect of air pollution on a population depends on the pollution's chemical makeup. The U.S. Environmental Protection Agency (EPA) lists six "criteria pollutants" frequently monitored by state and local governments.[5] One of these pollutants is small particulate matter (PM), which is measured as having an aerodynamic diameter of less than 10 μm (PM_{10}) or less than 2.5 μm ($PM_{2.5}$). $PM_{2.5}$ may be more hazardous to human health than PM_{10} because it is small enough to bypass the clearance mechanisms in the nose and lung, enter the lower lung (alveoli), and even cross into the bloodstream.[1] $PM_{2.5}$ is primarily composed of fuel combustion products, road dust, and crustal materials.[6]

High-pressure weather systems that occur during cold weather can create temperature inversions, wherein a layer of warm air traps cold air below.[7] In mountain valleys, this also traps PM in the cold air layer. During inversions, $PM_{2.5}$ levels can exceed 100 μg/m^3 for several days, which is approximately triple the maximum EPA limits for healthy human exposure in a 24-hour period.

Cache County, Utah, is located in a large valley north of Salt Lake City along the Idaho border. The area is prone to inversions and home to Utah State University, mountains, fishing, and farmland.

▶ Case Study

Stage 1: Identifying a Need

Cache County health officials suspected that air pollution was a growing problem, so they began monitoring air pollution levels in the year 2000. They designated locations for large, stationary outdoor air pollution monitors that could continuously detect and collect PM. Each week, the Utah Department of Environmental Quality, Division of Air Quality (UDAQ), used the monitors to collect and analyze PM samples at 1-hour intervals. Over time, they acquired a lot of data (**FIGURE 4-1**).[8]

In December 2006, EPA designated a new 24-hour limit for $PM_{2.5}$; it dropped from 65 to 35 μg/m³ of air. EPA began reviewing data from across the country to identify counties that needed help meeting the new limit. Cache County sent the $PM_{2.5}$ data it had acquired to UDAQ and EPA to determine if the county had attained the designated levels (Figure 4-1).

Stage 2: Policy Development

Josh Greer,*[9] the environmental health director for the Bear River Health Department in Logan, Cache County, returned to his office after a meeting with the county council. In accordance with the new $PM_{2.5}$ limit, and using the data supplied

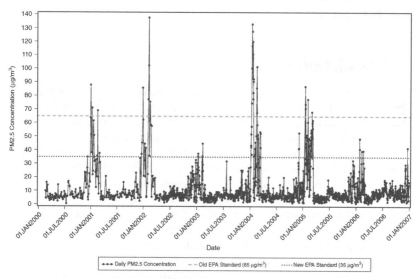

FIGURE 4-1 24-hour mean Cache County $PM_{2.5}$ levels from 2000 to 2006.

Abbreviations: EPA, U.S. Environmental Protection Agency; $PM_{2.5}$, particulate matter smaller than 2.5 μm.

U.S. Environmental Protection Agency. (2017). Air data: Air quality data collected at outdoor monitors across the US. Retrieved from https://www.epa.gov/outdoor-air-quality-data

---

* Mr. Greer has given permission for his name to be used.

by UDAQ, EPA had designated Cache County as being in "non-attainment" on December 14, 2009. It was now 2011. The county decided to delegate the authority to mitigate the $PM_{2.5}$ problem to the Bear River Health Department.

Due to the non-attainment designation, Utah was required to prepare a State Implementation Plan (SIP) by December 14, 2012. The SIP had to detail initiatives for meeting the new $PM_{2.5}$ limit by 2014. UDAQ worked with Cache County to develop policies that would help reduce its $PM_{2.5}$ problem. Josh worked with statisticians, who reviewed the data and developed statistical models to determine the largest sources of $PM_{2.5}$. They found that about 50% of $PM_{2.5}$ in the air came from motor vehicles.

EPA does not require motor vehicle emissions testing. Emissions programs are designated by states based on their individual circumstances. Unlike every other state that requires emissions testing, per Utah Code Section 41-6a-1642, vehicle emissions programs required under federal law (as part of the SIP) are to be developed and operated by the legislative body of the non-attainment county rather than by the state. Josh and his team decided that because motor vehicles were by far the most prominent sources of $PM_{2.5}$, emissions testing would need to be a major part of the SIP going forward.

The work moved forward rapidly. Cache County needed to implement a program quickly to attain the federal $PM_{2.5}$ limit and avoid penalties such as the withholding of highway maintenance funds. However, it encountered many barriers. Not all county council members were receptive to emissions testing, and it took several meetings to convince some members. Members of the community who drove older vehicles and farming equipment also worried that the new regulations placed an unfair burden on them. Josh went back and forth between the county officials and the statisticians for months. The statisticians tested dozens of scenarios under which different types of vehicles would need to meet various standards. The county wanted to minimize the burden of the regulations, but still meet its attainment goals.

In 2012, the Cache County Council voted on ordinance 2013-04, which failed to pass. After much discussion with state officials and EPA, the ordinance finally passed on March 12, 2013, and delegated the county's authority to the Bear River District Board of Health to "address all issues pertaining to the adoption and administration of the vehicle emission inspection and maintenance program."

While the health department was seeking approval for an emissions program, the Metropolitan Planning Organization (MPO) for Utah received funds each year from the federal government to reduce $PM_{2.5}$ levels in Cache County. The MPO knew that an emissions testing program was on the horizon, so it saved the funds so that additional funds would not be needed to launch the program.

Josh worked closely with an associate from UDAQ who was "on loan" to help the Bear River Health Department. Josh had already been actively designing an emissions program in the hope that it would receive approval so that it could move forward. Josh visited different emissions programs, talked with vendors, and went back and forth with the county council members. He came up with a plan that, based on his research, should reduce emissions without being overly burdensome for typical automobile drivers.

On May 9, 2013, Josh received approval to move forward with his plan: Vehicles less than 7 years old would not have to be tested, but vehicles 7 years old or older would have to undergo emissions testing every other year and the standards would be based on the weight of the vehicle.

Types of emission tests included onboard diagnostics (OBD), two-speed idle (TSI), and diesel tampering. For OBD tests, testers would connect to vehicles' onboard computers and communicate with them to validate that appropriate driving conditions had been met, required sensors had run, and no emissions-related faults had been identified. These inspections would be performed on light-duty gasoline vehicles (1996 and newer, up to 8500 lb), medium-duty gasoline vehicles (2008 and newer, up to 14,000 lb), and diesel vehicles (2007 and newer, up to 14,000 lb). For TSI tests, pollutants that came from vehicles' tailpipes would be measured at a high speed (2200–2800 revolutions per minute [RPM]) and an idling speed (350–1100 RPM). Standards would be based on vehicles' model year and weight. Older gasoline-powered vehicles (1995 and older) and heavier gasoline-powered vehicles (more than 14,000 lb) would receive a TSI test. For diesel tampering tests, required emissions control devices would be searched for and inspectors would ensure that the devices were in place and apparently operable. Diesel vehicles (1998–2006, up to 14,000 lb) would be tested by this method.

Stage 3: Policy Implementation and Evaluation

Josh had from May 9, 2013, to January 1, 2014, to implement the emissions program. He had to recruit an equipment vendor, set up a system for recruiting and training mechanics, and actively communicate the new requirements to the public. Normally, recruiting a vendor alone could take up to 2 years.

On July 3, 2013, the Bear River Health Department released a Request for Proposals (RFP) from vendors. A committee of five people not involved in the program design was chosen to review proposals so that the process of choosing a vendor would remain unbiased. They set a proposal due date of August 12, 2013, and received a good response. The committee reviewed the proposals quickly, and on August 27, 2013, selected Worldwide Environmental Products (Brea, CA), to provide equipment.

Josh then went to work developing training for mechanics. He worked with Worldwide Environmental Products to test equipment and develop administrative procedures. Working at a frenzied pace, emission tests began by December, and the program officially launched January 1, 2014.

Cache County, UDAQ, and EPA all monitored data regarding Cache County's $PM_{2.5}$ levels over the next few years (**TABLE 4-1**).[8] Meanwhile, other air pollution mitigation efforts increased. For example, there were efforts to reduce emissions from paint, newer vehicles with better smog ratings became available, new fuel standards were implemented, and there was an increased effort to reduce vehicle idling.

The program tested the emissions of more than 46,000 vehicles in its first year (**TABLE 4-2**).[8] Evaluating the effectiveness of Josh's program would be essential to determine whether it could and should continue, what funds could be appropriated to it, and most importantly, whether it was having a positive impact on the $PM_{2.5}$ levels and health of people in Cache County (**TABLE 4-3**).[10]

TABLE 4-1 Summary Statistics for 24-Hour Mean County-Level PM$_{2.5}$ in January and February 2014–2017

	2014	2015	2016	2017	4-Year Average
Mean	17.3	10.2	18.1	18.7	15.9
Standard deviation	15.1	7.2	12.3	19.2	8.1
Minimum	3.1	1.7	0.9	1	2.5
5th percentile	4.2	2.5	2.8	1.4	4.1
10th percentile	4.5	3	4.6	1.9	4.8
Quartile 1	5.7	4.7	7.6	3.5	8.8
Median	8.9	8.2	16.9	11.6	14.6
Quartile 3	27.9	15.9	26.2	27.1	22.1
90th percentile	42.9	22.8	35.9	43.3	27.2
95th percentile	45.4	23.2	39.2	60.1	28.4
Maximum	49	28.3	46.8	84.7	31.5
Total number of exceedances of new EPA limit (35 μg/m³) (%)	13 (22)	0 (0)	8 (13)	12 (20)	8.3 (14)

Abbreviations: EPA, U.S. Environmental Protection Agency; PM$_{2.5}$, particulate matter smaller than 2.5 μm.

U.S. Environmental Protection Agency. (2017). Air data: Air quality data collected at outdoor monitors across the US. Retrieved from https://www.epa.gov/outdoor-air-quality-data

Summary Points

1. Small airborne particulate matter (PM) is dangerous to the health of individuals, especially if they have preexisting health conditions, are very young, or are older than 65 years.
2. Cache County, Utah, collected air quality data to determine if it had a problem with PM air pollution; using these data, the U.S. Environmental Protection Agency (EPA) designated Cache County as in "non-attainment" of the PM limit.

TABLE 4-2 Total Number of Inspections and Failures for Different Vehicle Types in Cache County by Year

Year	Total OBD Inspections	Total OBD Failures	Total TSI Inspections	Total TSI Failures	Total Tampering Inspections	Total Tampering Failures
2014	36,103	6324	8677	2654	1302	45
2015	37,235	5849	8169	2643	1251	49
2016	40,126	5284	7156	1718	1349	49
2017	37,528	5002	6589	1465	1152	36

Abbreviations: OBD, onboard diagnostics; TSI, two-speed idle.

U.S. Environmental Protection Agency. (2017). Air data: Air quality data collected at outdoor monitors across the US. Retrieved from https://www.epa.gov/outdoor-air-quality-data

TABLE 4-3 Age-Adjusted Rates of ED Visits for Asthma and Myocardial Infarction in Cache County, 2006 and 2014

Health Outcome	Year	Number of ED Visits	Number in Population	Age-Adjusted Rate per 10,000[a]	95% CI	
Asthma	2006	154	101,236	15.61	13.06	18.51
	2014	149	118,177	11.98	10.04	14.18
Myocardial infarction	2006	51[b]	33,912[b]	7.75	5.76	10.20
	2014	102[b]	42,049[b]	12.06	9.82	14.67

Abbreviations: CI, confidence interval; ED, emergency department.
[a] Standardized to the U.S. population in 2000.
[b] Only individuals older than age 34 are included.

Data from Center for Health Data and Informatics, Utah Department of Health. (2017). Public Health Indicator Based Information System (IBIS): Utah's public health data resource. Retrieved from https://ibis.health.utah.gov/

3. The Bear River Health Department in Cache County, Utah, used the air quality data to develop a motor vehicles emissions program in response to the non-attainment designation by EPA.
4. The Bear River Health Department continues to use data to evaluate the effectiveness of this program.

▶ Application of CEPH MPH Competencies

This case study addresses CEPH competency 4.

Competency 4: Interpret Results of Data Analysis for Public Health Research, Policy, or Practice

Public health policies are ideally developed because a weight of evidence suggests the policy is needed and that it will be effective. However, there can be a disconnect between policy-makers and those individuals who collect, analyze, and interpret data. Persons who are in a position to formulate policy should understand how to read analytic results, such as tables and graphs, and draw correct conclusions from them. They also need to understand how to identify the limitations of certain data, what biases influence collection and analysis, and what factors may confound results. Students who become fluent in reading analytic results will be able to make policy-level decisions in their careers that are more beneficial to a larger group of people. They will also be able to explain the results of data analysis to the policy-makers with whom they interact.

When making policy decisions, data are often employed at multiple levels and across partnerships. As the results of data analysis are communicated to various groups, it is important to acknowledge that each group or entity may view the data differently through the lens of its own goals and values. If the scope and limitations of the data are not explicitly communicated, then decision making can be misled. Students must be able to ask objective questions about data sources, collection and analytic methods, and presentation of results to avoid these pitfalls.

As policies evolve, they must be continually evaluated. It can be difficult to identify which data to collect, and by which method, to inform continued decision making. Students need to be able to ask questions regarding data that are presented to them, so that they can move projects and policies forward in a positive direction in ways that continue to be based on evidence. This is the nature of the application of data to public health research, policy, and practice.

Discussion Questions

1. What was the main issue that Josh and his colleagues were trying to overcome?
2. What role did data collection and analysis play in determining whether Cache County had a particulate matter air pollution problem?
3. What role did data collection and analysis play in the development of Cache County's motor vehicle emissions program?
4. Based on the data, was the program effective? Why or why not?
5. What further data could Josh and his team collect to better understand the strengths and weaknesses of their program, its overall effectiveness, and potential changes (if needed)?

References

1. Pope, C. A. III, & Dockery, D. W. (2006). Health effects of fine particulate air pollution: Lines that connect. *Journal of the Air & Waste Management Association, 56*, 709–742.
2. Nel, A. E., Diaz-Sanchez, D., & Li, N. (2001). The role of particulate pollutants in pulmonary inflammation and asthma: Evidence for the involvement of organic chemicals and oxidative stress. *Current Opinion in Pulmonary Medicine, 7*, 20–26.
3. Brauer, M., Hoek, G., Val Vilet, P., Meliefste, K., Fischer, P. H., Wijga, A., … Brunekreef, B. (2002). Air pollution from traffic and the development of respiratory infections and asthmatic and allergic symptoms in children. *American Journal of Respiratory and Critical Care Medicine, 166*, 1092–1098.
4. Pope, C. A., Burnett, R. T., Thurston, G. D., Thun, M. J., Calle, E. E., Krewski, D., & Godleski, J. J. (2004). Cardiovascular mortality and long-term exposure to particulate air pollution: Epidemiological evidence of general pathophysiological pathways of disease. *Circulation, 109*, 71–77.
5. Suh, H. H., Bahadori, T., Vallarino, J., & Spengler, J. D. (2000). Criteria air pollutants and toxic air pollutants. *Environmental Health Perspectives, 108*, 625.
6. Wilson, W. E., & Suh, H. H. (1997). Fine particles and coarse particles: Concentration relationships relevant to epidemiologic studies. *Journal of the Air & Waste Management Association, 47*, 1238–1249.
7. Beard, J. D., Beck, C., Graham, R., Packham, S. C., Traphagan, M., Giles, R. T., & Morgan, J. G. (2012). Winter temperature inversions and emergency department visits for asthma in Salt Lake County, Utah, 2003–2008. *Environmental Health Perspectives, 120*, 1385.
8. U.S. Environmental Protection Agency. (2017). Air data: Air quality data collected at outdoor monitors across the US. Retrieved from https://www.epa.gov/outdoor-air-quality-data
9. Greer, J. (2018). Personal communication.
10. Center for Health Data and Informatics, Utah Department of Health. (2017). Public Health Indicator Based Information System (IBIS): Utah's public health data resource. Retrieved from https://ibis.health.utah.gov/

Public Health and Healthcare Systems

CHAPTER 5

Comparing Organizational Structure and Function of Healthcare and Public Health Systems: The Q5C Model for Quality, Coverage, Cost, Choice, Coordination, and Context

Scott H. Frank, MD, MS

Matthew Kucmanic, MPH, MA

▶ Background

In a dynamically changing health environment, it is useful to have a structure with which to evaluate changes in healthcare and public health systems within the United States and other global settings. The Q5C Model describes both domains and metrics to achieve this comparison, examining Quality, Coverage, Cost, Choice, Coordination, and Context for health systems. While these domains are interrelated, each offers important understanding of how to assess health systems. This case study allows students to apply this approach to three different healthcare systems from around the world and to rank the most effective system.[1]

Quality: What Outcomes Does the System Produce?

"The US healthcare system does not provide consistent, high quality medical care to all people."[2] This observation by the Institute of Medicine in 2001 represented a stark wake-up call to healthcare leadership. Health quality is defined as "the degree to which health care services for individuals and populations increase the likelihood of desired health outcomes and are consistent with current professional knowledge."[3] The most effective metrics for healthcare system quality involve health outcomes such as healthy lives (mortality amenable to healthcare interventions), infant mortality, life expectancy, and premature death. In addition, patient satisfaction and patient safety are key quality measures. Patient satisfaction is sometimes out of touch with evidence-based evaluations of quality, with patients rating their health system as more effective than the evidence supports.[4] Patient safety is assessed through tracking medical errors—communication breakdowns, diagnostic errors, poor judgment, and inadequate skill—and violations of patient safety are the third leading cause of death in the United States.[5]

Coverage: How Many People Are Covered? How Effective Is the Coverage? Does Coverage Promote Access to Health Care?

Coverage in the United States is primarily driven by private health insurance (67.5%), most of which is employer based (55.7%).[6] Government insurance is the next most common source of insurance (37.3%), consisting of both the Medicaid (19.4%) and Medicare (16.7%) programs. The uninsured rate has decreased by nearly half since the initiation of the Patient Protection and Affordable Care Act (ACA), from 16.3% in 2010 to 8.6% in 2016.[5] Uninsurance rates in 2016 remained higher for Hispanics (16%), Blacks (10.5%), and Asians (7.6%) than for non-Hispanic Whites (6.3%). When considering coverage access to care, availability of primary care, prevention services, and poor prescription coverage must be taken into account. Lack of insurance or access to primary care providers contributes to overuse of emergency rooms and to the increased cost of health care.

Cost: What Does the System Cost the Country? The Individual?

The cost of health care in the United States is by far the highest cost found anywhere in the world. The United States spent $3.3 trillion on health care in 2016, or 17.9% of the gross domestic product (GDP). The annual cost of health care has risen from $146 per person in 1960 to $10,348 in 2016. As much as 30% of U.S. healthcare spending does not contribute to improvement of individual or population health.[7] The primary contributors to high healthcare costs appear to be more testing and treatments ordered by clinicians and higher prices for those products and services.[8] U.S. hospital prices, for example, are 60% higher than those in Europe.[9] High administrative costs and the fee-for-service payment approach also contribute substantially to the high U.S. healthcare costs.[10] It is important to note that illness rates are not responsible for the increase in healthcare spending: Indeed, the higher the quality of care, the lower the healthcare spending.[6] Chronic diseases such as diabetes and heart disease account for 85% of healthcare costs and are largely preventable through primary and secondary prevention, which might be achieved through public health spending. Healthcare costs involve not only costs to society but also the personal consequences of rising health insurance cost, out-of-pocket medical expenses, and medical bankruptcy.

Choice: Is There Freedom for Individuals to Choose Their Doctors, Testing, and Treatment? Is There Freedom for Clinicians to Choose?

In many ways, freedom of choice defines U.S. values, expressed in health care as the opportunity and autonomy to act without constraint by others. These values drive the persistence of private insurance healthcare model in the United States, which seeks to maximize—with limitations—freedom to choose your doctor, medical treatments and procedures, and medications. Government or single-payer plans, it is assumed, will decide for you and limit choice, which is considered decidedly "un-American." However, choice in the United States is often limited by availability, geography, out-of-pocket cost, forced discontinuity, and inability to pay. Thus, freedom to choose health care is available to those who can afford such freedom, but even then is limited by cost-reducing limitations imposed by health insurers. Paradoxically, consumer-driven choice does not lead to greater efficiency or higher quality in health care but rather has a negative impact on health equity.[11] Choice also extends to clinicians' capacity to choose what they believe is the best testing or treatment for patients, a hallmark of the U.S. health system that is increasingly limited by restrictions imposed by insurance and administrative restrictions.[12] Metrics for choice include the latitude to choose your own physician; access to generalist, preventive, emergency, and specialty care; restrictions of services or pharmaceuticals; availability of procedures; and long wait times.

Coordination: Is the Healthcare System Effectively Coordinated? Is There Coordination Between Medicine and Public Health?

Coordination of care among healthcare providers has been described as the single most important criterion for patient satisfaction.[13] In the United States, just 25% of health plans provide coordination of care among doctors and other healthcare providers. Fragmentation has been described as "the heart of the ineffectiveness of our increasingly frantic efforts to nurture improvement."[14] Fragmentation is associated with inefficiency, ineffectiveness, commoditization, commercialization, deprofessionalization, depersonalization, and dissatisfaction.

There is an equally urgent need for coordination between medicine and public health. In the United States, public health spending represents less than 5% of overall healthcare spending. Further, medical spending is inversely related to public health spending.[15] Yet in areas with higher public health spending, there are significant reductions in mortality,[16] whereas increases in medical spending are not related to improved health outcomes or patient satisfaction.[17] In fact, patient satisfaction has been shown to increase with greater public health spending and to decrease with higher private health spending and the availability of more hospital beds.[18] Coordination can be assessed through effectiveness of communication among healthcare providers.

Context: Is Importance Placed on Conditions Conducive to Good Health?

Context refers to the world outside of health care. When examining contributors to premature death, inadequate health care offers only a 10% contribution, whereas 30% of these contributions is attributed to genetic predisposition. Context accounts for the other 60%, including 40% relating to behavior patterns, 15% to social circumstances, and 5% to environmental exposure.[19] Context represents society's contribution to the well-being of its citizens through social spending, primary prevention, and health promotion. Countries that spend more on social welfare programs have better health outcomes.[20]

Health occurs in the context of place and daily life. The ecology of health care[21] points out that only 22% of people who develop health symptoms engage with the healthcare system, with only 0.1% becoming hospitalized. Context involves the 78% of people each month who experience symptoms but are not patients, who receive no direct benefit from the $267 billion spent per month on health care in the United States. Assessment of context can be achieved through measures of health equity, public health funding, social spending, and social determinants of health such as under-education, racial segregation, social support, and poverty.[21]

▶ Case Study

This case study describes three international healthcare systems and provides information necessary to assess their quality, coverage, cost, choice, coordination, and context. As you evaluate these systems, rank them and try to identify the county involved.

Country A

In Country A, most employed people under the age of 65 share premiums for a group health insurance policy with their employer. The insurance company picks up most of the cost, with the patient making copayments. If a person loses a job, health insurance is lost as well. Numerous for-profit health insurance corporations offer group insurance policies. Individuals whose employers do not offer group health insurance coverage may purchase health insurance as individuals, albeit at a higher cost. The health insurance companies may choose to insure or not insure an individual and set the cost based on age, health history, gender, and preexisting conditions. People over the age of 65 and the poor receive coverage through government health insurance plans. The uninsured have access to medical care if they can pay out of pocket or if they are sick enough to be admitted to a public hospital. When the uninsured must receive substantial medical care, the bills may result in personal bankruptcy.

Country A's public health system utilizes only 4% of national health expenditures and is ranked 15th among the world's best public health systems. Country A ranks last in care effectiveness, efficiency, and safety, and has 21% underuse of recommended medical care because of its cost. Health expenditures represents 17.9% of the country's GDP. Infant mortality is 6.4/1000 live births; life expectancy is 76 years for men and 81 years for women; mortality amenable to health care is 110 deaths per 100,000 population. Wait times are longest for primary care and emergency care, but shortest for specialty services. Country A ranks first on provision of clinical preventive services, yet ranks last in terms of health equity and long, productive, healthy lives.

Country B

In Country B, healthcare payers, providers, clinics, and hospitals are private entities. Country B uses private, nonprofit health insurance plans paid for jointly by employers and employees through payroll deductions that are a flat percentage of wages, with more than 100 plans to choose from. Regardless of the plan, people pay the same amount and receive the same benefits. Everyone must belong to a plan. For those not employed, the government subsidizes the cost of coverage.

Country B has the world's third best public health system. It ranks third in care effectiveness, second in efficiency, and second in safety. Country B has 15% underuse of recommended medical care because of its cost. Health expenditures represent 11.3% of the country's GDP. Infant mortality is 3.6/1000 live births; life expectancy is 78 years for men and 83 years for women; mortality amenable to health care is 76 deaths per 100,000 population. Country B ranks last in provision of preventive service, but is tied for the best ranking on healthcare equity. Wait times are typically short; on a global scale, they rank shortest for emergency care and for elective or non-emergency surgery, and second shortest for primary care and for specialty services. Country B ranks first in terms of its population having long, productive, healthy lives.

Country C

In Country C, health care is provided and financed by the government through tax payments. Hospitals and clinics are largely owned by the government. Doctors may be government employees or have private practices, but all collect their fees from the government. Country C has low costs per citizen because the government controls which services doctors can be reimbursed for and the levels of reimbursements, focusing on evidence-based coverage of tests and treatment.

Country C ranks first in care effectiveness, efficiency, and safety, and has only 4% underuse of recommended medical care because of cost. Patients pay nothing when they receive medical care, because health care is considered a public service in the same way as fire departments or public libraries. Country C ranks second in preventive care and has the world's fourth best public health system. Health expenditures represent 9.4% of the country's GDP. Infant mortality in Country C is 4.3/1000 live births; life expectancy is 78 years for women and 82 years for men; mortality amenable to health care is 83 deaths per 100,000 population. Wait times are short for primary care and emergency care, but long for elective or non-emergency surgery and specialty services. Country C ranks second in provision of preventive services, but first in terms of healthcare equity. Country C ranks second for long, productive, healthy lives.

Summary Points

1.   Healthcare systems differ by quality, coverage, cost, choice, coordination, and context as a result of each country's unique social, cultural, historical, and political realities.
2.   Healthcare coverage is a hallmark of a fair and equitable healthcare system. From the perspective of public health, it is crucial and ethical to ensure that all people are given full access and that a lack of individual resources should not determine healthcare decisions.
3.   Analysis of health systems is often exclusive to health care and does not consider the crucial role of context and community-based prevention, which are strongly influenced by public health.

▶ Application of CEPH MPH Competencies

This case study addresses CEPH competency 5.

Competency 5: Compare the Organization, Structure, and Function of Health Care, Public Health, and Regulatory Systems Across National and International Settings

Analysis of the organization, structure, and function of health care and public health systems is best accomplished through use of a comprehensive, structured approach. This application allows discernment across relevant components of each system, generating integrated understanding. Among these three countries, the United Kingdom ranks first, followed by Germany, and then the United States.

Country A: United States 2010 (Pre-ACA)

Quality: WHO Health System Ranking 37/37. Poorest patient safety. Highest mortality for causes amenable to health care.

Coverage: Poorest access to care as a result of a large uninsured population.

Cost: High cost to consumers; high cost to government; high pay to physicians, especially specialists.

Coordination: Poorest in coordination of care. Poorest communication between specialists and primary care.

Choice: Shorter waits for specialty care and elective procedures; longer for emergency and primary care. Good choice for both consumers and physicians among the insured. Timeliness of care ranked last.

Context: Poor health equity largely a result of uninsurance and damaging social determinants of health. Moderate community prevention, best clinical prevention.

The assessment of the U.S. healthcare system improved in quality, coverage, and coordination in 2014 after partial implementation of the ACA. There was no change in cost, choice, or context. The United States still ranked last overall among healthcare systems.[3]

Country B: Germany

Quality: WHO Health System Ranking 25/37. Ranks high on patient safety, effective care, and patient-centered care. Second best mortality for causes amenable to health care.

Coverage: Universal coverage, most consistent access across health sectors.

Cost: Low cost to consumers; low cost to government; lowest pay to specialty physicians.

Coordination: Lowest in coordinated care.

Choice: Best balance of short waits for emergency, and primary, and specialty care, and for elective procedures. Good choice for both consumers and physicians. Timeliness of care ranked second.

Context: Strong health equity. Moderate community prevention; moderate clinical prevention.

Country C: United Kingdom

Quality: WHO Health System Ranking 18/37. Best effectiveness and safety. Conflicting findings, with second worst mortality for causes amenable to health care.

Coverage: Universal coverage.

Cost: Lowest cost to consumers; lowest cost to government. Active proof that high-quality care costs less. Moderate pay to physicians; smallest difference between specialty and primary care.

Coordination: Ranked first among these countries in coordination of care.

Choice: Short waits for emergency and primary care. Long waits for specialty care and elective procedures. Fewest options available for both consumers and physicians. Timeliness of care best.

Context: Highest health equity. Moderate community prevention; moderate clinical prevention.

Discussion Questions

1. In which health system would you personally prefer to receive health care? Why?
2. Which three components of the Q5C model are most important to you personally? Which might be most important to your parents or grandparents? Why?
3. This analysis focused on the U.S. health system in 2010, before the ACA was passed. How might this analysis change while the ACA was functioning? How do you think it might evolve in the future?

References

1. Reid, T. R. (2010). *The healing of America: A global quest for better, cheaper, and fairer health care*. London, UK: The Penguin Press.
2. Institute of Medicine. (2001, March). *Crossing the quality chasm: A new health system for the 21th century*. Washington, DC: National Academies Press. https://doi.org/10.17226/10027
3. Davis, K., Stremikis, K., Squires, D., & Schoen, C. (2014). *Mirror, mirror on the wall: How the performance of the US health care system compares internationally*. New York, NY: The Commonwealth Fund. Retrieved from https://www.commonwealthfund.org/sites/default/files/documents/___media_files_publications_fund_report_2014_jun_1755_davis_mirror_mirror_2014.pdf
4. Blendon, R. J., Kim, M., & Benson, J. M. (2001). The public versus the World Health Organization on health system performance. *Health Affairs, 20*(3), 10–20. https://doi.org/10.1377/hlthaff.20.3.10
5. Makary, M. A., & Daniel, M. (2016). Medical error-the third leading cause of death in the US. *BMJ*. https://doi.org/10.1136/bmj.i2139
6. Barnett, J. C., & Berchick, E. R. (2017). Health insurance coverage in the United States: 2016. *Current Population Reports*, 60–260.
7. Tran, L. D., Zimmerman, F. J., & Fielding, J. E. (2017). Public health and the economy could be served by reallocating medical expenditures to social programs. *SSM: Population Health, 3*, 185–191. https://doi.org/10.1016/J.SSMPH.2017.01.004
8. Dieleman, J. L., Squires, E., Bui, A. L., Campbell, M., Chapin, A., Hamavid, H., . . . Murray, C. J. L. (2017). Factors associated with increases in US health care spending, 1996-2013. *Journal of the American Medical Association, 318*(17), 1668. https://doi.org/10.1001/jama.2017.15927
9. Koechlin, F., Lorenzoni, L., & Schreyer, P. (2010). *Comparing price levels of hospital services across countries: Results of pilot study*. OECD Health Working Papers, No. 53. Paris, France: OECD Publishing. http://dx.doi.org/10.1787/5km91p4f3rzw-en
10. Spiro, T., Lee, E. O., & Emanuel, E. J. (2012). Price and utilization: Why we must target both to curb health care costs. *Annals of Internal Medicine, 157*(8), 586. https://doi.org/10.7326/0003-4819-157-8-201210160-00014
11. Fotaki, M. (2013). Is patient choice the future of health care systems? *International Journal of Health Policy and Management, 1*(2), 121–123. https://doi.org/10.15171/ijhpm.2013.22
12. Gawande, A. (2009). The cost conundrum. *The New Yorker*. Retrieved from https://www.newyorker.com/magazine/2009/06/01/the-cost-conundrum
13. J. D. Power. (2017). Health plan satisfaction driven by coordination of care with providers, *J.D. Power* finds. Retrieved from https://www.prnewswire.com/news-releases/health-plan-satisfaction-driven-by-coordination-of-care-with-providers-jd-power-finds-300463599.html
14. Stange, K. C. (2009). The problem of fragmentation and the need for integrative solutions. *Annals of Family Medicine, 7*(2), 100–103. https://doi.org/10.1370/afm.971
15. Mays, G. P., Smith, S. A., Ingram, R. C., Racster, L. J., Lamberth, C. D., & Lovely, E. S. (2009). Public health delivery systems. *American Journal of Preventive Medicine, 36*(3), 256–265. https://doi.org/10.1016/j.amepre.2008.11.008

16. Mays, G. P., & Smith, S. A. (2011). Evidence links increases in public health spending to declines in preventable deaths. *Health Affairs (Project Hope), 30*(8), 1585–1593. https://doi.org/10.1377/hlthaff.2011.0196

17. Fisher, E. S., Wennberg, D. E., Stukel, T. A., Gottlieb, D. J., Lucas, F. L., & Pinder, É. L. (2003). The implications of regional variations in Medicare spending. Part 1: The content, quality, and accessibility of care. *Annals of Internal Medicine, 138*(4), 273. https://doi.org/10.7326/0003-4819-138-4-200302180-00006

18. Xesfingi, S., & Vozikis, A. (2016). Patient satisfaction with the healthcare system: Assessing the impact of socio-economic and healthcare provision factors. *BMC Health Services Research.* https://doi.org/10.1186/s12913-016-1327-4

19. McGinnis, J. M., Williams-Russo, P., & Knickman, J. R. (2002). The case for more active policy attention to health promotion. *Health Affairs, 21*(2), 78–93. https://doi.org/10.1377/hlthaff.21.2.78

20. Stuckler, D., Basu, S., & McKee, M. (2010). Budget crises, health, and social welfare programmes. *BMJ (Clinical Research Education), 340*, c3311. https://doi.org/10.1136/BMJ.C3311

21. Green, L. A., Fryer, G. E., Yawn, B. P., Lanier, D., & Dovey, S. M. (2001). The ecology of medical care revisited. *New England Journal of Medicine, 344*(26), 2021–2025. https://doi.org/10.1056/NEJM200106283442611

CHAPTER 6

Centering Wellness: Using Black Feminist Literature as a Public Health Pedagogical Tool for Personal Healing, Community Health, and Social Justice

LeConté J. Dill, DrPH, MPH

▶ Background

Students often come to public health classrooms and learning spaces embodying anxiety, depression, and stress, and carrying the responsibility of familial and community obligations. Stressors evolve from such demands that are made by the internal or external environment and that upset homeostasis.[1] Such psychosocial stressors are actually fueled by inequities stemming from structural and societal oppressions, such as racism, sexism, heterosexism, classism, and ableism.[2] Scholars, activists, and scholar-activists have provided language, analyses, and tools to understand and address the "interlocking systems of oppression" of racism, sexism, heterosexism, classism, and ableism.[3-5] These systems of oppression have been identified as having a central role in the production and reproduction of health inequalities.[6,7]

These systems of oppression that go on to manifest as psychosocial stressors are biophysiologically incorporated into our bodies—a notion illuminated by the epidemiologic concept of embodiment.[8,9] Our pervasive awareness and vigilant responses to these stressors begin to cause "wear and tear" onto our bodies.[10] Trauma results from experiencing an event, a series of events, or a set of circumstances that are physically or emotionally harmful or life threatening.[11] Systemic oppressions contribute to acute trauma in individuals and chronic trauma within communities.[11] Trauma can have a significant impact on the development, health, and well-being of individuals, families, and communities.[11]

Fortunately, the effects of trauma can be addressed and retraumatization can be prevented through healing-centered engagement.[12] Such a healing-centered engagement involves a centering of wellness principles, pedagogies, and practices. People exposed to the aforementioned trauma are not solely the victims of that trauma; they have the agency to center their own wellness and that of their communities.

▶ Case Study

This case study offers lessons and learnings from the master of public health–level "Centering Wellness" course, which was first introduced at the State University of New York (SUNY) Downstate School of Public Health. For public health professionals, the aforementioned intersecting oppressions do not just manifest externally in society and in the lives of our patients, clients, and community partners. That is, dominant hegemonic practices are also embedded in traditional approaches to public health curricula, which tend to downplay the primacy of racism, sexism, heterosexism, classism, and ableism in our lives.[13,14] The Centering Wellness course offers a pedagogical space to promote health and manage the effects of illness, stress, and trauma. As public health professionals, our focus is inherently on the health of "the public," oftentimes at the expense or erasure of our own individual health. This notion was captured by poet, novelist, and activist Asha Bandele: "tho we constantly lose our footing trying to heal a world before healing ourselves first."[15] In this same vein, the Centering Wellness course is premised on the following questions:

1. How does embodiment impact how we pursue, practice, and advocate for greater community health and wellness?

2. How do classroom spaces, class discussions, and academic culture and expectations increase students' stress and anxiety, particularly when their daily realities and stressors are not acknowledged or addressed?

The Centering Wellness course explores the adage from the 1960s second-wave Feminist movement, "The personal is political," and what this saying means for learners and practitioners of public health. Specifically, this course engages multigenre works written by women of African descent over the past 50 years that have inspired and/or make up Black Feminist theory and praxis to explore how their characters experience illness and trauma and how they engage in multiple practices of healing and recovery. Such experiences in literature can serve as rich examples for emerging health professionals to critically examine their own analysis and role in engendering personal and collective healing, health, and wellness in the understanding and pursuit of social justice. The Black Feminist epistemological and pedagogical approaches underlying the Centering Wellness class are aimed at supporting students in interrogating the intersecting oppressions of racism, sexism, heterosexism, classism, and ableism,[4,5] while also working to combat such oppressions that fuel personal and community health inequities. Black Feminist foremother Patricia Hill Collins[4] consistently reminds us that U.S. Black women generate social theory to combat such intersecting oppressions. Black feminist theory, in the form of poetry, fiction, music, visual art, or essays, is at times intentionally divergent from hegemonic academic textual forms.[4]

In the novel *The Salt Eaters*, Black Feminist writer, teacher, and scholar Toni Cade Bambara,[16] through her character Minnie, asks the protagonist Velma: "Are you sure, sweetheart, that you want to be well?" (p. 3), then follows that inquiry with an admonition: "Just so's you're sure, sweetheart, and ready to be healed, cause wholeness is no trifling matter. A lot of weight when you're well" (p. 10). In the midst of systemic degradation and oppression,[17] the Centering Wellness students are called to unpack and pursue this notion of wholeness-as-wellness.

As a decolonial and Black Feminist pedagogical practice,[18] students in the Centering Wellness class are named and treated as "co-learners" alongside the instructor. This commitment is informed by Black Feminist scholar Bell Hooks's[19] transgressive, transformative, and engaged pedagogy. She states:

> Making the classroom a democratic setting where everyone feels a responsibility to contribute is a central goal of transformative pedagogy... . Accepting the decentering of the West globally, embracing multiculturalism, compels educators to focus attention on the issue of voice. Who speaks? Who listens? And why? (pp. 39–40)

As co-learners, the students and instructor of the Centering Wellness course engage in "mutual vulnerability,"[20] completing the same assignments, which may stretch their comfort zones, but work to reveal themselves more fully. To engage in such mutual vulnerability, as the first assignment in the course, co-learners are invited to create a "Femifesto"[21]— a public declaration of their beliefs and visions. Specifically, learners are asked to detail what kind of public health practitioner or scholar they are and want to be. Furthermore, at the end of each week, learners are invited to write in an online journal (or a hardcopy journal or notebook) a few sentences to a paragraph responding to the following question: *How did I honor myself this week?* If learners are engaged in social media and willing to share these reflections, they are asked to use the hashtag #WhenIFellInLoveWithMyself. The prompt and hashtag comes from women's health scholar-activist Barlow[22] and her applied research related to mental health and well-being for Black women, in which participants upload digital videos responding to the same and related prompts.

The structure of the Centering Wellness course is organized around a socio-ecological perspective of illness and wellness. Critical reading assignments consist of poetry, fiction, memoir, plays, and ethnography written by Black women that delve into topics such as structural violence, intergenerational trauma, intimate-partner violence, cancer, HIV/AIDS, and suicide, but also spiritual health, self-discovery, recovery, and resilience. In the first iteration of the Centering Wellness course in the spring of 2017, some of the authors with which participants engaged included the Combahee River Collective, Dr. Mary Weems, Anna Deavere-Smith, Dr. Bettina Judd, Sonia Sanchez, Audre Lorde, Mahogany Browne, Helena Andrews, Toni Morrison, and Octavia Butler.

Additionally, the teaching methods and structure of the Centering Wellness course align with contemplative practices and principles of contemplative pedagogy, which connect students' lived, embodied experiences to their own learning.[23] Meditation, visualization, music, dance, and storytelling are woven directly into the Centering Wellness curriculum, as informed by contemplative pedagogy. Through such approaches, students become more reflective of their sense of purpose, feel less anxious, and are enabled to explore their creativity. Additionally, students deepen their critical thinking skills.

Furthermore, we engage in methods of auto-ethnography[24] and performance ethnography[25] to connect the theoretical content and insights of the class with public health praxis. To this point, Hooks[19] states:

> The quest for knowledge that allows us to unite theory and practice is one such passion. To the extent that professors bring this passion, which has to be fundamentally rooted in a love for ideas we are able to inspire, the classroom becomes a dynamic place where transformations in social relations are concretely actualized. (p. 195)

The creation of wellness collages, body maps, affirmations, hashtags, blogs, poems, monologues, songs, and choreography represent Centering Wellness co-learners' pursuit of knowledge and can serve as their roadmap to wellness.

Although Centering Wellness was first taught as a semester-long master's-level course, versions of the course have been conducted as community workshops, trainings for staff at community-based organizations, and presentations at professional conferences. Additionally, undergraduate institutions and high schools have expressed interest in bringing the Centering Wellness course to their campuses.

Lessons learned from implementing the course are that instructors must consider the time and emotional intensity of completing the Centering Wellness activities alongside student co-learners. These activities are done while holding space for student emotions, healing, and learning, while also holding students accountable for course deliverables. Moreover, an expanded notion of course "evaluation" can result from implementing the Centering Wellness course, as "outcomes" and "impact" are much more expansive and contain a lot of rich narrative and emotive data.

Summary Points

1. Structural bias, social inequities, and racism contribute to stress, trauma, and ill health.
2. Black Feminist pedagogical practices illuminate systems of oppressions and opportunities for healing.

3. Reading, analyzing, and developing creative projects help public health learners to engage in multiple practices of healing and recovery.
4. Centering personal wellness better equips public health practitioners in combating health inequities.

▶ Application of CEPH MPH Competencies

This case study addresses CEPH competency 6.

Competency 6: Discuss the Means by Which Structural Bias, Social Inequities, and Racism Undermine Health and Create Challenges to Achieving Health Equity at Organizational, Community, and Societal Levels

Students begin the Centering Wellness course by reading and analyzing the Combahee River Collective Statement,[3] which helps them to understand and begin to critically discuss the impacts of the intersections of racism, sexism, heterosexism, classism, and ableism on society. These systems of oppression are fundamental causes for health inequities.[26] The students learn the notion of standpoint theory as articulated by the Combahee River Collective Statement—that our own individual perspectives are shaped by our social and political positioning in the world. In turn, students come to understand the importance of recognizing and understanding and articulating one's own standpoint and positionality while working collaboratively with diverse communities to achieve health equity. Students go on to create a Femifesto,[21] in which they detail their own standpoint and positionality regarding what kind of public health practitioner or scholar they are and want to be.

Structural bias creates differential opportunities along racial, gender, sexuality, socioeconomic, and physical ability lines.[26] Students in the Centering Wellness course continue to explore the impacts of structural bias on health by critically reading and analyzing public health literature that details societal inequities, racism, and historical trauma. Public Health Critical Race Praxis (PHCRP)[7] equips learners with a culturally relevant lens through which to analyze the impacts of structural bias on health. PHCRP moves "beyond documenting health inequities toward understanding and challenging the power hierarchies that undergird them."[7] Only by understanding and challenging these inequities can we individually and collectively amplify resilience and achieve equity.

To better understand the persistent social inequities that contribute to health inequities, students in the Centering Wellness course critically read and analyze creative works that explore the health impacts of structural violence, such as redlining, urban renewal, deindustrialization, and over-policing in communities.[27,28] Students also read and analyze creative works that explore chronic and infectious diseases,[29–31] as well as complementary public health research that details sexual, physical, mental, and emotional ill health. Then, students create body maps[32] so as to locate internal and external impacts upon their bodies. Using paper handouts of a body outline, as well as markers, crayons, key words, and phrases, these body maps enable students to qualitatively examine Krieger's concept of embodiment.[9]

As students begin to imagine the possibilities of dismantling systemic oppressions, combating persistent health inequities, and achieving health equity, they apply concepts garnered through the Centering Wellness course. Students critically read and analyze literature that delves into concepts such as cultural humility[33] and critical hope,[34] thereby considering culturally specific assets that might aid in creating more effective personal and community health interventions. Additionally, students create a Wellness Collage, in which they visually narrate their own personal illness, injury, recovery, and/or wellness story. Students critically read and analyze research-informed poetry that explores self-discovery, recovery, and healing.[35,36] Additionally, students engage in participatory narrative analysis,[37] wherein they write interpretive poems based on a topic from the course. Finally, students in the Centering Wellness course complete a group project, in which they creatively represent a wellness concern and strategies for disease prevention and health promotion.

Discussion Questions

1. How does Black Feminist theory and praxis apply to combating health inequities?
2. We tend to center "illness" in public health; what does it mean to center "wellness"?
3. What are some contemplative practices that can be applied in the public health classroom?
4. How can public health students benefit from engaging in creative projects?

▶ Acknowledgments

My deepest appreciation to the students in the spring 2017 Centering Wellness class at SUNY Downstate School of Public Health, who initially helped to activate this curriculum. Additionally, sincere thanks to Dr. Vivian Chávez, whose course "Promoting Positive Health" at San Francisco State University set a precedent for such courses and for such engaged and embodied pedagogy within our field of public health. A previous iteration of this case study was presented at the 2017 Hip Hop Literacies Conference in New York City.

References

1. Lazarus, R. S., & Cohen, J. B. (1977). Environmental stress. In I. Altman & J. F. Wohlwill (Eds.), *Human behavior and environment* (pp. 89–127). Boston, MA: Springer.
2. Marmot, M., & Wilkinson, R. (Eds.). (2005). *Social determinants of health*. Oxford, UK: Oxford University Press.
3. Combahee River Collective. (1977). "A black feminist statement." New York, NY: Kitchen Table: Women of Color Press.
4. Collins, P. H. (1990). *Black Feminist thought: Knowledge, consciousness, and the politics of empowerment*. Boston, MA: Unwin Hyman.
5. Crenshaw, K. W. (1991). Mapping the margins: Intersectionality, identity politics, and violence against women of color. *Stanford Law Review*, 43, 1241–1299.

6. Schulz, A. J., & Mullings, L. E. (2006). *Gender, race, class, and health: Intersectional approaches.* San Francisco, CA: Jossey-Bass.

7. Ford, C. L., & Airhihenbuwa, C. O. (2010). The public health critical race methodology: Praxis for antiracism research. *Social Science & Medicine, 71*(8), 1390–1398.

8. Krieger, N. (2001). Theories for social epidemiology in the 21st century: An ecosocial perspective. *International Journal of Epidemiology, 30*(4), 668–677.

9. Krieger, N. (2005). Embodiment: A conceptual glossary for epidemiology. *Journal of Epidemiology & Community Health, 59*(5), 350–355.

10. McEwen, B. S., & Seeman, T. (1999). Protective and damaging effects of mediators of stress: Elaborating and testing the concepts of allostasis and allostatic load. *Annals of the New York Academy of Sciences, 896*(1), 30–47.

11. Calvo, M., Ukeje, C., Abraham, R., & Libman, K. (2016). *Trauma-informed and resilient communities: A primer for public health practitioners.* New York, NY: New York Academy of Medicine.

12. Ginwright, S. A. (2015). Radically healing Black lives: A love note to justice. *New Directions for Student Leadership, 2015*(148), 33–44.

13. Airhihenbuwa, C. O. (1994). Health promotion and the discourse on culture: Implications for empowerment. *Health Education Quarterly, 21*(3), 345–353.

14. Wallerstein, N. (2006). What is the evidence on effectiveness of empowerment to improve health? *Health evidence network report* (pp. 1-37). Copenhagen, Denmark: WHO Regional Office for Europe.

15. Bandele, A. (1999). on the way out of san francisco i wrote this poem. In *absence in the palms of my hands* (p. 71). New York, NY: Harlem River Press.

16. Bambara, T. C. (1980). *The salt eaters.* New York, NY: Vintage.

17. Diaz, J., & Fullwood, S. G. (2014, November). The weight in being well: *The Salt Eaters* and the genius of Toni Cade Bambara. *The Feminist Wire.* Retrieved from https://thefeministwire .com/2014/11/weight-in-being-well/

18. Dill, L. J. (In press). #CrunkPublicHealth: Decolonial Feminist praxes of cultivating liberatory and transdisciplinary learning, research, and action spaces. In J. Ford & N. Jaramillo (Eds.), *Decolonial womanisms.* Champaign, IL: University of Illinois Press.

19. Hooks, B. (1994). *Teaching to transgress: Education as the practice of freedom.* New York, NY: Routledge.

20. Guishard, M. (2009). The false paths, the endless labors, the turns now this way and now that: Participatory action research, mutual vulnerability, and the politics of inquiry. *Urban Review, 41*(1), 85–105.

21. Brathwaite, B., & Ferrara, M. (2016). The Homegirl Box. Retrieved from https:// thehomegirlbox.com/our-story

22. Barlow, J. (2016). #WhenIFellInLoveWithMyself: Disrupting the gaze and loving our Black Womanist self as an act of political warfare. *Meridians: Feminism, Race, Transnationalism, 15*(1), 205–217.

23. Rendón, L. I., & Kanagala, V. (2017). Embracing contemplative pedagogy in a culturally diverse classroom. *Social Justice, Inner Work & Contemplative Practice, 1*(1), 15–25.

24. Boylorn, R. M., & Orbe, M. P. (2014). Critical autoethnography as a method of choice. In R. M. Boylorn & M. P. Orbe (Eds.), *Critical autoethnography: Intersecting cultural identities in everyday life* (pp. 13–26). Walnut Creek, CA: Left Coast Press.

25. Cox, A. M. (2015). *Shapeshifters: Black girls and the choreography of citizenship.* Durham, NC: Duke University Press.

26. Gee, G. C., & Ford, C. L. (2011). Structural racism and health inequities: Old issues, new directions. *Du Bois Review: Social Science Research on Race, 8*(1), 115–132.

27. Smith, A. D. (2003). *Twilight—Los Angeles, 1992.* New York, NY: Dramatists Play Service Inc.

28. Weems, M. E. (2011). *Closure.* Somerville, MA: Kattywompus Press.

29. Lorde, A. (1997). *The cancer journals: Special edition.* San Francisco, CA: Aunt Lute.

30. Sanchez, S. (1997). *Does your house have lions?* Boston, MA: Beacon Press.

31. Browne, M. L. (2015). *Redbone.* Detroit, MI: Willow Books.

32. Ruglis, J. (2011). Mapping the biopolitics of school dropout and youth resistance. *International Journal of Qualitative Studies in Education, 24*(5), 627–637.

33. Tervalon, M., & Murray-Garcia, J. (1998). Cultural humility versus cultural competence: A critical distinction in defining physician training outcomes in multicultural education. *Journal of Health Care for the Poor and Underserved, 9*(2), 117–125.

34. Duncan-Andrade, J. (2009). Note to educators: Hope required when growing roses in concrete. *Harvard Educational Review, 79*(2), 181–194.

35. Yancey, A. (1997). *An old soul with a young spirit: Poetry in the era of desegregation recovery: Self-discovery, social commentary, health advocacy.* Los Angeles, CA: Imhotep.

36. Judd, B. (2014). *Patient.* New York, NY: Black Lawrence Press.

37. Dill, L. J. (2015). Poetic justice: Engaging in participatory narrative analysis to find solace in the "Killer Corridor." *American Journal of Community Psychology, 55*(1–2), 128–135.

Planning and Management to Promote Health

CHAPTER 7

Using Participatory Methods to Create a Community Action Plan for a Rural Community Coalition

Nandi A. Marshall, DrPH, MPH, CHES
Lynn D. Woodhouse, EdD, MPH
John S. Luque, PhD, MPH
Gulzar H. Shah, PhD, MStat, MS
Cassandra Arroyo, PhD, MS

▶ Background

Community coalitions and partnerships have been an integral part of public health research and practice over the past 3 decades.[1,2] Coalition structure varies widely based on the purpose for which the coalition is formed. Ideally, community coalitions should have a broad representation of stakeholders—not only experts in government public health agencies, health care, research, nongovernmental organizations, and so on, but also a fair representation of community experts (i.e., residents, local organization leadership, business leaders, faith-based organization leadership). Coalition membership is a critical factor in establishing a baseline understanding of the local health issues and their determinants, which then serves as the foundation for community coalition action planning. Several methods could be employed to establish this baseline understanding, including qualitative methods such as photovoice and planning models like the Community Readiness Model.[3,4]

Photovoice is a process by which people can identify, represent, and enhance their community through a specific photographic technique. This method has traditionally entrusted cameras to the hands of people to enable them to act as recorders, and potential catalysts for change, in their own communities.[5] While the use of photovoice is not the focus of this case study, the results from a photovoice project were used to complement the data collected through implementation of the Community Readiness Model.

The Community Readiness Model consists of two main components created to guide community assessments and action planning. The first component is the community readiness assessment, which is completed through key informant interviews. These interviews, which focus on the six "dimensions of readiness for prevention," are then scored to determine the level of readiness for action in that surveyed community. The rating scales, detailed in the *Community Readiness Model Handbook*, quantify scores for each of the responses in six dimensions: community efforts, community knowledge of the efforts, leadership, community climate, community knowledge about the issue, and resources related to the issue.[6] The second component is brainstorming and action planning. Once the issues are selected, the community uses the brainstorming and action planning sessions to determine how they will address those issues by taking the readiness level score into consideration.[6,7]

The Community Readiness Model is designed to facilitate community change while integrating the culture of a community, the existing resources, and the level of readiness to support the efforts of community members in effectively addressing an issue.[3,4,8,9] This model is unique in its ability to address an array of issues, allow the community to define its own issues and strategies, and increase the community's capacity for prevention and intervention. In addition, the model can be used to assess the degree to which a community is ready to participate in change, and to guide the process of community change.[9-11]

While the first application of the Community Readiness Model was focused on drug and alcohol misuse among the American Indian population, the model can be applied to any community that can be defined by geography, an issue, or organization.[9,12,13] To date, the Community Readiness Model has been successfully used to intervene in childhood obesity,[4,11,14-16] understand rural community leaders' readiness for a leisure-based health promotion program in their town,[17] prevent sexual violence,[18] and assess community readiness to participate in a community-wide obesity prevention program.[19]

▶ Case Study

Located in rural southeast Georgia, the community coalition (at the time of this case study) was funded by the Society for Public Health Education (SOPHE) Health Equity Project through a partnership with Georgia Chapter of SOPHE. Assisting with the grant application, working closely with the ongoing coalition facilitator and the project coordinator, and having close contact with the coalition during its progression afforded the project lead a sense of rapport with the coalition. Due to the previous grants being solely focused on capacity building and infrastructure, the coalition members expressed an interest in participating in the creation of an action plan to address diabetes in their community. The coalition members were eager to contribute to an action planning process that would not only be informed by their opinions but also include other stakeholders in the community. In turn, the project lead presented some options that might be appealing to the group; these included photovoice and the Community Readiness Model. After engaging in discussions, the coalition voted to use these tools to inform their community coalition action plan. Institutional review board (IRB) approval was obtained before the methods were actually implemented.

Guided by the ecological perspective,[20] with a focus on expanding the understanding of the social determinants of health, this case study utilized the photovoice results and gathered additional qualitative data to explore the processes of community coalition action planning through the lens of the Community Readiness Model. Participants for the brainstorming/action planning and the in-depth interviews (and photovoice) were all active members in the community coalition. Its membership is made up of nurses, retired educators, local law enforcement, county elected officials, childcare providers, city government employees, and unemployed persons. The ages represented in the coalition range from 18 to 85 years, although the majority of the active members fell toward the higher end of the age range.

Informed consent forms were used throughout the data collection process, including the key informant interviews and the community coalition action planning process—both key pieces of the Community Readiness Model. Informed consent was also obtained for the members who participated in the photovoice component. While that process will not be discussed in depth in this case study, the results from the photovoice piece were included in the community coalition action planning. Participants were required to complete and sign the associated informed consent form for each corresponding activity to ensure they were fully aware of the associated risks.

In preparation for the key informant interview process, the community coalition recommended 10 members of the larger community, who were not directly associated with the coalition, to be considered. The coalition viewed these individuals as leaders in the community who might provide valuable insights into the community climate and available resources. These informants represented the fields of education, medicine, senior care, and clergy.

The Community Readiness Model provides potential questions for the key informant interviews, as well as a guide for brainstorming and action planning.[9]

Key Informant Interviews

A meeting with the ongoing coalition facilitator, the interim community coalition chair, and the project facilitator was held to determine the potential need for additional questions that might benefit the coalition's future activities. Two questions were added to the key informant survey: (1) How does your organization market (advertise) its services? and (2) Would you, or someone from your organization, be interested in serving on an advisory board for the County Diabetes Coalition? These questions were added to the existing set of interview questions provided by the Community Readiness Model and modified for applicability. The questions available through the Community Readiness Model have the capability of being adapted for any "issue" and, in this case, were edited to focus on diabetes prevention and management in the county. This information was used for the community readiness assessment and to provide contextual information for the action planning process.

After making initial contact with the recommended interviewees, appointments were scheduled with 8 of the 10 individuals. Two of the recommended informants declined the interview. One of informants' supervisors was also recommended to be a key informant and agreed to be interviewed. As a result, the decision was made by the supervisor and potential key informant to interview only the supervisor. The other informant expressed no knowledge about diabetes in the county and declined the interview. Six of the interviews were held in person, with two additional interviews held via separate phone calls. All of the interviews were recorded, transcribed, and entered into the qualitative software. The codes used to analyze these transcripts represented the areas measured in the interview:

- ECE: Existing community efforts
- CKE: Community knowledge of efforts
- L: Leadership
- CC: Community climate
- CKI: Community knowledge about the issue
- RDPM: Resources related to the issue (diabetes prevention and management)
- P: Prevention
- MISC: Miscellaneous

The "Prevention" and "Miscellaneous" categories were added during the coding process.

After coding, the information was transferred to a matrix word document to further examine the themes and quotes identified in the qualitative software. The transcripts were then assessed by two reviewers to identify the community readiness score for each interview. Interview responses, categorized by six "dimensions of readiness for prevention," were scored using a step-by-step process that yielded an overall readiness level for the county. The reviewers independently scored the interviews, compared and tallied the scores, and determined the community's readiness level, which was a 2.52.

This score falls within Stage 2 of the Community Readiness Model, which encompasses scores ranging from 2 to 3 points. Communities in this stage are identified by the model as being in denial or resisting the issue. This means that there is recognition of the issue as a problem, but no ownership of it has been taken as a local problem. Even with this recognition, there is a feeling that nothing needs to be done about it locally.[6] This perspective was apparent in some of the responses provided by the key informants. There was recognition of the need for a personal connection to understand that diabetes was a problem in the community and that the community was at risk. The readiness level contributed to the activities included in the community coalition action plan.[6]

Brainstorming and Action Planning

Information received from the photovoice project, the key informant interviews, and the readiness score were used to create the final action plan. Brainstorming and action planning began with brief summaries of the key informant interviews, the photovoice process and its results, and an overview and implications of the community readiness score. The themes presented were used as the starting point for the action plan. During the planning process, the project lead also facilitated a conversation focused on challenges and opportunities that were not previously identified by coalition members. In addition to activities focused on improving health in their community, the coalition members opted to include strategies to address those challenges and optimize the resources and opportunities. As the group discussed each challenge and resource, they also decided who should be reached, what would be provided to them, why this group was important, and how the coalition would make an impact.

The draft coalition action plan was created by synthesizing the notes from the planning session. The action plan was presented to and reviewed by the coalition. After a brief discussion of the action plan, the coalition adopted the community coalition action plan by a majority vote.

Summary Points

1. Participatory methods for assessing community needs, assets, and capacities, such as the Community Readiness Model, provide invaluable evidence and insights for community action planning around community health issues.
2. The Community Readiness Model is an appropriate tool to use in rural settings where quantitative survey methods are not as feasible to apply.
3. Brainstorming and action planning need to incorporate the community's views on the presence of social determinants contributing to or creating health inequities.
4. The application of participatory methods offers unique opportunities to demonstrate Council on Education for Public Health (CEPH) competencies across multiple categories.

▶ Application of CEPH MPH Competencies

Competency 7: Assess Population Needs, Assets, and Capacities that Affect Communities' Health

The focus of this case study was the process used in guiding a rural community coalition through an action planning process under the aegis of the Community Readiness Model. The purpose of this model is to guide communities through assessing needs, assets, and current capacity of the focal community. Through the key informant interviews, data were collected to provide a snapshot of the community's readiness to address diabetes prevention and management for its population. The interview questions explored the community's knowledge of current efforts to address diabetes, the leadership's views regarding this issue as it related to the county, the current community climate, the community's knowledge of the actual issue, and resources available for prevention and management, including current policies and practices.[6] The interview data, coupled with the data gathered from the photovoice activity, provided the foundation for the community coalition to create its community action plan.

Competency 4: Interpret Results of Data Analysis for Public Health Research, Policy, or Practice

The key informant interviews were analyzed by two researchers for content and thematic analysis using both qualitative data management software and matrices. These data were then used, along with the photovoice data, to inform the community coalition action planning process. The action plan was subsequently implemented by the coalition the following year.

Competency 6: Discuss the Means by Which Structural Bias, Social Inequities, and Racism Undermine Health and Create Challenges to Achieving Health Equity at Organizational, Community, and Societal Levels

As mentioned in the introduction, the framing for this case study was not just application of the ecological model but also the discussions during the action planning process with the interviewees and the coalition members, which focused on the social determinants of health. Given that the coalition's focus was diabetes, it was important to discuss the different ways that the lived environment affects health outcomes. Some of these ideas were displayed in the overview of the photovoice results; others were discussed during the actual planning sessions. There were rich discussions around access, education, and lack of resources in this southern rural county and how they affect the health outcomes of the county.

Competency 8: Apply Awareness of Cultural Values and Practices to the Design or Implementation of Public Health Policies or Programs

The members of the community coalition were almost all members of the community that they served. The majority of them, having belonged to the community for decades, had a unique understanding of the vast cultural values and practices of the community. They were able to convey those ideals and priorities within the action planning process. Having an action plan that not only represents the current needs of the community but also includes their values allows for greater community buy-in, participation, and support.

Discussion Questions

1. How does community ownership play a role in the success of action planning?
2. A community's immediate needs oftentimes outweigh overall public health needs. Using the Community Readiness Model, how would you approach addressing the community-identified priorities versus public health data trends, if different?
3. Select three levels of the ecological model and describe one strategy for each level that you would implement, based on the readiness score of this community, and explain why.

▶ Disclaimer

This project was supported by the Cooperative Agreement Number 5U58DP002328-05 from the Centers for Disease Control and Prevention (CDC). Its contents are solely the responsibility of the authors and do not necessarily represent the official views of the CDC.

References

1. Butterfoss, F. D., & Kegler, M. (2009). The community coalition action theory. In R. J. DiClemente, R. A. Crosby, & M. Kegler (Eds.), *Emerging theories in health promotion practice and research* (pp. 237–276). San Francisco, CA: John Wiley and Sons.
2. Winterbauer, N. L., Bekemeier, B., VanRaemdonck, L., & Hoover, A. G. (2016). Applying community-based participatory research partnership principles to public health practice-based research networks. *SAGE Open, 6*(4), 2158244016679211.
3. Crooks, V., Giesbrecht, M., Castleden, H., Schuurman, N., Skinner, M., & Williams, A. (2018). Community readiness and momentum: Identifying and including community-driven variables in a mixed-method rural palliative care service siting model. *BMC Palliative Care, 17*(1), 59.
4. Kesten, J. M., Cameron, N., & Griffiths, P. L. (2013). Assessing community readiness for overweight and obesity prevention in pre-adolescent girls: A case study. *BMC Public Health, 13*(1), 1205.
5. Wang, C., & Burris, M.A. (1997). Photovoice: Concept, methodology, and use for participatory needs assessment. *Health Education and Behavior, 24*(3), 369–387.
6. Plested, B. A., Edwards, R. W., & Jumper-Thurman, P. (2006). *Community readiness: A handbook for successful change.* Fort Collins, CO: Tri-Ethnic Center for Prevention Research.
7. Kelly, K. J., & Stanley, L. (2014). Identifying upstream factors using the community readiness model: The case of reducing alcohol use among college students. *Journal of Social Marketing, 4*(2), 176–191.
8. Edwards, R. W., Jumper-Thurman, P., Plested, B. A., Oetting, E. R., & Swanson, L (2000). Community readiness: Research to practice. *Journal of Community Psychology, 28*(3), 291–307.
9. Plested, B. A., Jumper-Thurman, P., & Edwards, R.W (2009). *Community readiness: Advancing "this issue" prevention in Native communities (Community readiness model manual, revised edition).* Fort Collins, CO: Ethnic Studies Department.
10. Jarpe-Ratner, E., Fagen, M., Day, J., Gilmet, K., Prudowsky, J., Neiger, B. L., . . . Flay, B. R. (2013). Using the Community Readiness Model as an approach to formative evaluation. *Health Promotion Practice, 14*(5), 649–655.
11. Hildebrand, D., Blevins, P., Betts, N., & Brown, B. (2015). Use of the Community Readiness Model to develop and evaluate a chef-based training program for school nutrition professionals. *Journal of Nutrition Education and Behavior, 47*(4), S28–S29.
12. Plested, B. A., Jumper-Thurman, P., Edwards, R. W., & Oetting, E. R. (1998). Community readiness: A tool for effective community-based prevention. *Prevention Researcher, 5*(2), 5–7.
13. Jumper-Thurman, P., Plested, B. A., Edwards, R. W., Helm, H. M., & Oetting, E. R. (2001). Using the Community Readiness Model in Native communities. In J. E. Trimble & F. Beauvais (Eds.), *Health promotion and substance abuse prevention among American Indian and Alaska Native communities: Issues in cultural competence* (CSAP Monograph, Cultural Competence Series No. 9, DHHS Publication No. SMA 99-3440, pp. 129–158). Rockville, MD: U.S. Department of Health and Human Services.
14. Findholt, N. (2007). Application of the Community Readiness Model for childhood obesity prevention. *Public Health Nursing, 24*(6), 565–570.
15. Frerichs, L., Brittin, J., Robbins, R., Steenson, S., Stewart, C., Fisher, C., & Huang, T. T. (2015). Peer reviewed: SaludABLEOmaha: Improving readiness to address obesity through healthy lifestyle in a Midwestern Latino community, 2011–2013. *Preventing Chronic Disease, 12.* doi: 10.5888/pcd12.140328

16. Kesten, J. M., Griffiths, P. L., & Cameron, N. (2015). A critical discussion of the Community Readiness Model using a case study of childhood obesity prevention in England. *Health & Social Care in the Community, 23*(3), 262–271.

17. Son, J. S., Shinew, K. J., & Harvey, I. S. (2011). Community readiness for leisure-based health promotion: Findings from an underserved and racially diverse rural community. *Journal of Park and Recreation Administration, 29*(2), 90–106.

18. Duma, S., & De Villiers, T. (2016). Community Readiness Model for prevention of sexual violence on campus in South Africa. Presentation given at the 27th International Nursing Research Congress. *Virginia Henderson Global Nursing e-Repository.* Retrieved from https://sigma .nursingrepository.org/handle/10755/616480

19. Sliwa, A., Goldberg, J. P., Clark, V., Collins, J., Edwards, R., Hyatt, R. R., . . . Economos, C. D. (2011). Using the Community Readiness Model to select communities for a community-wide obesity prevention intervention. *Preventing Chronic Disease, 8*(6), 1–9.

20. Harris, M. (2010). *Evaluating public and community health programs.* San Francisco, CA: Jossey Bass.

CHAPTER 8

Adapting an Evidence-Based, Sexual Risk Reduction Intervention to Be More Inclusive of Trans and Cis Girls

Elizabeth A. Baker, PhD, MPH, CPH

▶ Background

Despite national, state, and local efforts to improve sexual health outcomes, sexually transmitted infections (STIs) and unintended pregnancy continue to disproportionately affect youth and young adults in the United States.[1,2] According to the Centers for Disease Control and Prevention (CDC), young people age 15 to 24 years account for 50% of new STI cases, yet represent only one-fourth of sexually active individuals.[1] Further disparities are documented among young, sexually active females[a]—one in four reports an STI diagnosis. Likewise, while teen pregnancy rates are at an all-time low, rates remain substantially higher in the United States than those documented in other Western, industrialized nations.[2,3] Moreover, persons born female who identify as a gender or sexual minority (e.g., lesbian, bisexual, transgender, or queer) appear to be at greater risks for STIs and

---

a The terms *female(s)* and *male(s)* in this chapter are defined by extant literature and data collection instruments that equate female(s) and male(s) to persons identified as *female-bodied* or *male-bodied*, respectively, at birth. Their use is not endorsed by the author, who recognizes the transmisogyny of the terms and definitions.

pregnancy compared to their straight, cis-gender peers (defined as persons whose gender identity matches the sex that they were assigned at birth)—a public health topic that remains grossly understudied.[4] The existing literature suggests that these outcomes result from a mix of biological, behavioral, and cultural factors, as briefly summarized here.

Biological Factors

Biologically, females are more susceptible to STIs than males due to cervical ectopy (i.e., columnar cells found in the cervical canal, located on the outer surface of the cervix).[1] Although these cells are common in adolescent and young adult females, they are more susceptible to invasion by STIs. As normal development of the reproductive system continues, the process of metaplasia (i.e., transformation of one differentiated cell type to another) transforms the columnar cells (i.e., soft cells) into squamous cells (i.e., hard cells).[5] Accordingly, as females age, cervical ectopy decreases, as does the risk of infection.

Behavioral Factors

Excluding the use of reproductive technologies, such as in vitro fertilization, pregnancy may occur when an ovulating female has unprotected vaginal–penile intercourse with a male who has adequate sperm levels for fertilization.[4] While this behavior is often conceptualized as an interaction between a straight, cis-gender male and female, research suggests that sexual behavior is not always concordant with sexual orientation, desire, or attraction. In fact, a mounting body of research suggests that youth who identify as sexual or gender minorities are more likely than their straight, cis-gender peers to report ever having vaginal sex, early sexual initiation (defined as sexual penetration before age 13 or 14 years), more frequent vaginal sex, more sexual partners, and unprotected sex.[4,6] While reasons for these observations remain unclear, several studies suggest that these youth are more likely to have sex under the influence of drugs and alcohol and/or to be victims of sexual violence, including homophobic or transphobic bullying. Likewise, youth who identify as sexual or gender minorities disproportionately account for youth in foster care, homeless youth, and runaways—all of whom report higher rates of unintended pregnancy and STIs, in general. Furthermore, these youth are less likely to report being influenced by protective factors, including family support, social acceptance among peers, and school connectedness (defined as "a sense of belonging and being part of school along with feeling cared about by teachers and other school staff" [p. 163]).[4]

Cultural Factors

While a few cultural and environmental factors that contribute to higher STI and pregnancy rates among youth who identify as sexual or gender minorities were previously mentioned, several more warrant discussion.[6] For example, prevention programs historically have been tailored to straight youth, with the underlying assumption that youth who identify as sexual or gender minorities are not vulnerable. Consequently, curriculum may use gendered terms such as *boyfriend* instead of *sexual partner*. Moreover, youth may be present in different environments, including school and work, where anti-bullying and harassment policies inclusive of sexual orientation and gender identity and expression may be nonexistent, weak, or unenforced. Likewise, authentic representations of sexual and gender minorities remain underrepresented in the media, and few healthcare providers have received training or continued education related to caring for this subpopulation of persons, in general.

▶ Case Study

The Health Improvement Project for Teens (*HIP Teens*) is one of the most recent, evidence-based interventions recognized by the U.S. Department of Health and Human Services' (HHS) Office of Adolescent Health (OAH) for teen pregnancy prevention (TPP), as well as the CDC for human immunodeficiency virus (HIV) and STI prevention.[7,8] A positive youth development program, *HIP Teens* is the only brief evidence-based intervention with a high study rating (designated by the HHS's Teen Pregnancy Prevention Evidence Review) that includes post-intervention booster sessions. According to HHS, *HIP Teens* also impacts more behavioral outcomes than most interventions identified by the OAH, including (1) recent sexual activity, (2) number of sexual partners, (3) frequency of sexual activity, and (4) contraceptive use and consistency.[8,9]

Development of HIP Teens

HIP Teens was developed through extensive community-based participatory research (CBPR), in response to the notable absence of evidenced-based, gender-specific interventions available for community and clinic-based settings.[9-15] As such, the program was designed to reduce sexual risk behavior among adolescent females, age 15 to 19 years, and consists of four 2-hour sessions (totaling 8 hours), an intervention time that developers determined to be relevant, realistic, and reproducible, as well as scientifically validated for outcomes. In addition, two 90-minute booster sessions (totaling 3 hours) are delivered 3 and 6 months after the initial program.[9,11] Thus, the intervention includes six total sessions.

Theoretical Framework

HIP Teens is theoretically guided by a prominent theoretical framework, the Information–Motivation–Behavioral Skill (IMB) model, which suggests that social-cognitive variables such as knowledge, attitudes, social norms, and interpersonal skills predict sexual risk prevention behavior.[16,17] The constructs in the IMB model have accounted for most of the variance explaining these prevention behaviors that is modifiable and, therefore, forms the foundation for many effective interventions with diverse populations and age groups.[16,18]

Specifically, in the context of sexual risk reduction, the IMB model suggests that sexual risk reduction is determined by the extent to which people have the requisite knowledge, motivation, and skills to engage in risk reduction behaviors. Several studies, including the *HIP Teens* efficacy trial, have supported the theoretical links in this framework, which hypothesizes that information and motivation are partially mediated by behavioral skills to influence the initiation and maintenance of healthy sexual behaviors.[17,19]

In the *HIP Teens* curriculum, the informational component provides medically accurate, age-appropriate information on teen pregnancy, STI/HIV infection, and risk reduction strategies. Likewise, the motivational component specifically focuses on (1) helping participants understand why changing their risky behaviors is desirable and (2) building a commitment to health behavior change. Concerns that influence both immediate (behavior-focused) and broader-based motivation related to life goals, personal and community values, and other trans-situational influences within a gender-specific context are presented. Lastly, the behavioral skills component focuses on communicating assertively, improving self-efficacy, negotiating condom use and other safer sex practices with partners, and identifying high-risk situations.[16,17]

The Data

In the *HIP Teens* randomized controlled trial (RCT), 738 sexually active urban adolescent females were recruited from diverse community settings in a mid-size northeastern U.S. city.[9] The participants were randomized either to the *HIP Teens* intervention or to a structurally equivalent health promotion control group. Assessments and behavioral data were collected using audio computer-assisted self-interview (ACASI) at baseline, then at 3, 6, and 12 months post intervention.[9,20] Use of ACASI led to increased valid and reliable reports of risk behaviors.[20] Major behavioral findings of the RCT are outlined in **TABLE 8-1**.

TABLE 8-1 Major Behavioral Findings of the HIP Teens Randomized Controlled Trial

Outcomes	Post Intervention		
	3 Months	6 Months	12 Months
HIP Teens participants reported significantly fewer episodes of vaginal sex compared to control participants.	X	X	X
HIP Teens participants reported fewer incidence of unprotected vaginal sex compared to control participants.	X		X
HIP Teens participants reported a decrease in the number of sexual partners compared to control participants.	X	X	X
HIP Teens participants reported significant increases in sexual abstinence compared to control participants.			X

In addition, the research team could access and conduct patient chart audits for approximately two-thirds of the sample. With comparable numbers from both the intervention and controls groups audited, the research team identified a 50% reduction in positive pregnancy tests in the *HIP Teens* intervention group as compared to their control counterparts.[3]

Summary Points

1. *HIP Teens* seeks to reduce sexual risk behaviors among sexually active adolescent girls by increasing knowledge of HIV/STIs, increasing motivation to reduce sexual risk, and providing behavioral skill development, including negotiation, communication, decision-making, and condom-use skills.
2. This evidence-based intervention is theoretically driven by the Information–Motivation–Behavioral Skills (IMB) model.
3. Intervention methods are continually reviewed to ensure that the activities and content are culturally and developmentally appropriate, inclusive of LGBTQ (lesbian, gay, bisexual, transgender, questioning) participants, trauma informed, and medically accurate.

▶ Application of CEPH MPH Competencies

In 2015, the case study author, who maintains a research program focused on the reproductive justice of youth who identify as sexual or gender minorities, collaborated with the principal investigator of the *HIP Teens* RCT to enhance the curriculum to be more inclusive of trans and cis girls. This case study addresses CEPH competencies 8 and 19.

Competency 8: Apply Awareness of Cultural Values and Practices to the Design or Implementation of Public Health Policies or Programs

In this application, the researchers considered the *culture* of youth who identify as sexual and gender minorities. Importantly, the researchers recognized that not only are youth who identify as lesbian, gay, bisexual, or transgender separate groups but also that each of these groups encompasses subpopulations with their own unique health needs (based on race, ethnicity, socioeconomic status, geographic location, age, and other factors). At the same time, the researchers adopted the point of view expressed by the 2011 Committee on Lesbian, Gay, Bisexual, and Transgender Health Issues and Research Gaps and Opportunities: "the main commonality across these diverse groups is their members' historically marginalized social status relative to society's cultural norm of the exclusively heterosexual individual who conforms to traditional gender roles and expectations. Put another way, these groups share the common status of 'other' because of their members' departures from heterosexuality and gender norms" (p. 13).[21]

HIP Teens is designed to progress from practicing basic skills to more complex topics, including building social norms and drawing on participants' experiences.

Given the varying perspectives and life experiences of trans and cis girls, training and language were inserted into the *HIP Teen* training materials and implementation kits, respectively, to stress the importance of moderators reflecting on their own *implicit* or *explicit biases* (defined as the negative evaluation of one group and its members relative to another)[22] and moderating sessions with *cultural humility* (defined as a stance toward understanding culture; it requires a commitment to life-long learning, continuous self-reflection on one's own assumptions and practices, comfort with "not knowing," and recognition of the power/privilege imbalance that exists between clients and health professionals).[23] As such, moderators were encouraged to approach participants and group discussions with an openness to learn; to ask questions, rather than make assumptions; and to strive to understand, rather than to inform. While this approach was historically endorsed, it now was further situated in the context of implicit bias and cultural humility.

Likewise, moderators were encouraged to enforce similar "ground rules" for participants engaging in group discussions to best create a safe space for all. Specifically, moderators were encouraged to listen for *microaggressions* (defined as "subtle forms of discrimination, often unconscious or unintentional, that communicate hostile or derogatory messages, particularly to and about members of historically marginalized social groups"[24]) and to invite participants to "unpack" their use rather than dismiss them as a misunderstanding, a joke, or lack of "political correctness."

Competency 19: Communicate Audience-Appropriate Public Health Content, Both in Writing and Through Oral Presentation

In this context, public health content included the *HIP Teens* two-day training materials for moderators, the implementation kit (including the facilitator's guide and classroom PowerPoints), and the student workbook.

Heteronormative language is a cultural phenomenon in which language, in part, aligns with biological sex, sexuality, gender identity, and gender roles.[25] It is often associated with heterosexism, homophobia, and transmisogyny. Moreover, *identity-first language* is a type of linguistic prescription that may marginalize or dehumanize individuals by categorizing persons by a condition or identity (e.g., "an HIV patient" versus "a patient living with HIV") rather than as an individual or group of people who have that condition or identity.[26] As part of the 2015 *HIP Teens* adaptation, unintentional heteronormative and identity-first language used in the original RCT protocols and contents was replaced with more inclusive language, including *people-first language*,[b] guided by several language guidelines.[27-29] These required modifications to program methods, including games, interactive group activities, video clips, and role plays.

---

[b]   The author acknowledges and appreciates the use of identity-first language among persons who share that specific identity. It is important to note that, for some people, identity-first language is about a shared community, culture, and pride. Using identity-first language may be an intentional approach to embracing diversity and countering perceptions that certain identities are inherently negative. Use of identity-first versus people-first language remains controversial among health professionals.

Discussion Questions

1. To effectively demonstrate Competencies 8 and 19, public health professionals must be aware of their own implicit biases. Visit the *Project Implicit* website (https://implicit.harvard.edu/implicit/research/) to explore your potential biases and reflect on how they may impact your public health practice or research.
2. Consider a specific population you are interested in working with (or work with already). What are the linguistic practices of (1) persons who share that health condition or identity and (2) health professionals who provide services to that population? Would you (or do you) use identity-first or people-first language? Explain.
3. In this case study, a review of the literature informed the adaptation of an evidence-based, sexual risk reduction intervention to be more inclusive of youth who identify as sexual or gender minorities. Considering Competency 2, which other quantitative and/or qualitative data collection methods might a public health professional use to better adapt this curriculum for this subpopulation or other populations of interest? (*Hint*: Consider the formative research conducted to inform the original development of *HIP Teens*.)
4. How might a public health professional evaluate the adaptation of this intervention?

References

1. Centers for Disease Control and Prevention. (2017). *Sexually transmitted disease surveillance 2016*. Atlanta, GA: U.S. Department of Health and Human Services.
2. Martin, J. A., Hamilton, B. E., Osterman, M. J. K., Driscoll, A. K., & Drake, P. (2018). Births: Final data for 2016. *National Vital Statistics Reports, 67*(1). Hyattsville, MD: National Center for Health Statistics.
3. Sedgh, G., Finer, L. B., Bankole, A., Eilers, M. A., & Singh, S. (2015). Adolescent pregnancy, birth, and abortion rates across countries: Levels and recent trends. *Journal of Adolescent Health, 56*(2), 223–230. doi:10.1016/j.jadohealth.2014.09.007
4. Saewyc, E. M. (2014). Adolescent pregnancy among lesbian, gay, and bisexual teens. In A. Cherry & M. Dillon (Eds.), *International handbook of adolescent pregnancy* (pp. 159–169). Boston, MA: Springer.
5. Mazur, Y., & Pyrohova, V. (2018). Analysis of complicated cervical ectopy clinical course and recurrence. *Eureka: Health Sciences, 1*, 17–26. doi:10.21303/2504-5679.2018.00563
6. Office of Adolescent Health. (2015). Understanding LGBTQ youth & ensuring inclusivity in teen pregnancy prevention programs. Retrieved from https://www.hhs.gov/ash/oah/sites/default/files/ash/oah/oah-initiatives/assets/tpp-grantee-orientation/understanding-lgbtq-youth.pdf
7. Office of Adolescent Health. (2016). Health Improvement Project for Teens (*HIP Teens*). Retrieved from https://www.hhs.gov/ash/oah/grant-programs/teen-pregnancy-prevention-program-tpp/evidence-based-programs/hip-teens/index.html
8. Centers for Disease Control and Prevention. (2015). Health Improvement Project for Teens (*HIP Teens*). Retrieved from https://www.cdc.gov/hiv/pdf/research/interventionresearch/compendium/rr/cdc-hiv-hipteens_rr_good.pdf
9. Morrison-Beedy, D., Jones, S. H., Xia, Y., Tu, X., Crean, H. F., & Carey, M. P. (2013). Reducing sexual risk behavior in adolescent girls: Results from a randomized controlled trial. *Journal of Adolescent Health, 52*(3), 314–321. doi:10.1016/j.jadohealth.2012.07.005
10. Morrison-Beedy, D., Carey, M. P., Aronowitz, T., Mkandawire, L., & Dyne, J. (2002). Adolescents' input on the development of an HIV risk reduction intervention. *Journal of the Association of Nurses in AIDS Care, 13*(1), 21–27.

11. Morrison-Beedy, D., Carey, M. P., Crean, H. F., & Jones, S. H. (2011). Risk behaviors among adolescent girls in an HIV prevention trial. *Western Journal of Nursing Research, 33*(5), 690–711. doi:10.1177/0193945910379220

12. Morrison-Beedy, D., Carey, M. P., Crean, H. F., & Jones, S. H. (2010). Determinants of adolescent female attendance at an HIV risk reduction program. *Journal of the Association of Nurses in AIDS Care, 21*(2), 153–161. doi:10.1016/j.jana.2009.11.002

13. Morrison-Beedy, D., Carey, M. P., Kowalski, J., & Tu, X. (2005). Group-based HIV risk reduction intervention for adolescent girls: Evidence of feasibility and efficacy. *Research in Nursing & Health, 28*(1), 3–15.

14. Morrison-Beedy, D., Passmore, D., & Carey, M. P. (2013). Exit interviews from adolescent girls who participated in a sexual risk-reduction intervention: Implications for community-based health education promotion for adolescents. *Journal of Midwifery & Women's Health, 58*(3), 313–320. doi:10.1111/jmwh.12043

15. Seibold-Simpson, S., & Morrison-Beedy, D. (2010). Avoiding early study attrition in adolescent girls: Impact of recruitment contextual factors. *Western Journal of Nursing Research, 32*(6), 761–778.

16. Fisher, J., & Fisher, W. A. (1992). Changing AIDS-risk behavior. *Psychological Bulletin, 111*(3), 455–474.

17. Fisher, J. D., Kimble, D. L., Fisher, W. A., & Malloy, T. E. (1996). Changing AIDS risk behavior: Effects of an intervention emphasizing AIDS risk reduction information, motivation, and behavioral skills in a college student population. *Health Psychology, 15*(2), 114–123.

18. Fisher, J., & Fisher, W. A. (2000). Theoretical approaches to individual-level change in HIV risk behavior. In R. DiClemente (Ed.), *Handbook of HIV prevention* (pp. 3–56). New York, NY: Kluwer Academic/Plenum.

19. St. Lawrence, J. S., Brasfield, T. L., Jefferson, K. W., Alleyne, E., O'Bannon, R. E., & Shirley, A. (1995). Cognitive-behavioral intervention to reduce African American adolescents' risk for HIV infection. *Journal of Consulting and Clinical Psychology, 63*(2), 221–237.

20. Morrison-Beedy, D., Carey, M. P., & Tu, X. (2006). Accuracy of audio computer-assisted self-interviewing (ACASI) and self-administered questionnaires for the assessment of sexual behavior. *AIDS & Behavior, 10*(5), 541.

21. Institute of Medicine. (2011). *The health of lesbian, gay, bisexual, and transgender people: Building a foundation for better understanding*. Washington, DC: National Academies Press.

22. Blair, I., Steiner, J., & Havranek, E. (2011). Unconscious (implicit) bias and health disparities: Where do we go from here? *Permanente Journal, 15*(2), 71–78.

23. Tervalon, M., & Murray-Garcia, J. (1998). Cultural humility versus cultural competency: A critical distinction in defining physician training outcomes in multicultural education. *Journal for Health Care for the Poor and Underserved, 9*(2), 117–125.

24. Nadal, K., Whitman, C., Davis, L, Erazo, T., & Davidoff, K. (2016). Microaggressions toward lesbian, gay, bisexual, transgender, queer, and genderqueer people: A review of the literature. *Annual Review of Sex Research, 53*(4–5), 488–508.

25. Leap, W. (2007). Language, socialization, and silence in gay adolescence. In K. Lovaas & M. Jenkins, *Sexualities and communication in everyday life: A reader* (pp. 95–106). Thousand Oaks, CA: Sage.

26. Dunn, D., & Andrews, A. (2015). Person-first and identity-first language: Developing psychologists' cultural competence using disability language. *American Psychologist, 70*(3), 255–264.

27. Movement Advancement Project & GLAAD. (2012). An ally's guide to terminology: Talking about LGBT people & equality. Retrieved from http://www.glaad.org/sites/default/files/allys-guide-to-terminology_1.pdf

28. Human Rights Campaign. (2018). Glossary of terms. Retrieved from https://www.hrc.org/resources/glossary-of-terms

29. National LGBT Health Education Center. (2016). Glossary of LGBT terms for health care teams. Retrieved from https://www.lgbthealtheducation.org/wp-content/uploads/LGBT-Glossary_March2016.pdf

CHAPTER 9

Radon, the Silent Killer: Colorless, Odorless, But Forever Present Within Us

Elizabeth Squires, MPH, MCHES
David Milen, PhD

▶ Background

There are many concerns in public health (stroke, heart attack, diabetes, and cancer, for example), but one concern that has been garnering more attention in recent times is radon. In 1900, Dorn discovered the emanation from uranium that eventually became known as ^{222}Rn gas.[1] Radon can decay within 3 to 4 days, and can be found in rock, soil, groundwater, and other building materials. Lung cancer was found to be a key health indicator in those who were exposed to this type of inert gas for extended periods of time.[2] Further research by Dorn and scientists demonstrated that the gas was found in tap water and also caused high rates of cancer in coal miners. Studies continued to evolve in the 1920s and 1930s pertaining to incidence rates of cancer related to radon. It was found that the slow decay of radon materials eventually created by alpha radiation doses led to some of the major issues surrounding respiratory infections.[1]

During the 1950s and 1960s, further research was conducted by the Biological Effects of Ionizing Radiation Committee (BEIR Committee). Its BEIR Committee Report VI included various epidemiologic studies pertaining to a number of different coal mines. Of the 60,000 miners who had participated in the study, approximately 2600 miners had developed lung cancer. Later, studies in the late 1990s and early 2000s indicated high incidence rates of lung cancer due to the materials being used for housing and urban development.[1] Today, radon is the leading cause of lung cancer in nonsmokers, and the second leading cause of cancer overall, especially in the United States, due to the duration of exposure to radon that may be present in water, soil, building materials, or other materials.[2-4]

Exposure to hazardous materials, such as radon, has been linked to different types of cancer, infertility, sleep disturbances, and increased risk of asthma. Currently, air pollutants within homes often exceed the health standards regarding both chronic and acute exposures.[5] Most U.S. families spend approximately 90% of their daily lives indoors. Thus, the decay of radon products within residencies and work-related buildings can increase their health risks on a daily basis.[6]

Research has indicated there is a lack of information and educational opportunities for family members to learn about the health impacts of radon. In many instances, it was demonstrated that many people were ambiguous to the facts regarding radon as well as the impacts it could have upon their health. In some cases, residents and family members or acknowledge the fact that there may be radon within their residencies, but refuse to believe that any health side effects or health impacts would be likely stem from their exposure to it.[7]

▶ Case Study

In March 2017, a public health program at a university was contacted by the Environmental Protection Agency (EPA), Region 5, looking to complete a project with a local university and a city under the College/Underserved Community Partnership Program (CUPP). The purpose of this project was to increase the amount of radon testing in rental properties located within city limits. Two deliverables were requested: an ordinance proposal to mandate the testing of radon in rental properties located within the city and a health communication campaign on radon.

A Memorandum of Understanding (MOU) was drafted and signed between the EPA, Region 5, the city, and the university in April 2017.

The members of the Region 5 EPA, several members from the state as well as elected officials from the state, and many local area stakeholders were instrumental in moving the research project forward. Several meetings between students, professors, and the aforementioned stakeholders were needed to arrange how the research would be performed without compromising community relations between landlords and other community members. Due to the location of all stakeholders involved in the research, several conference calls were initiated weekly in an effort to collaborate both at the university level with students and by arranging meetings and presentations with community stakeholders. One meeting each week was initialized for approximately 6 months in an effort to maintain communication between all stakeholders. Occasionally, face-to-face meetings were needed to demonstrate updated information pertaining to the study, answer questions from stakeholders, and establish next steps for the project to move forward.

In May 2017, a total of 13 graduate public health students were recruited to help complete the project. Two full-time faculty members acted as project leads.

In June 2017, the students researched and wrote a community description of the city, using data from the U.S. Census to describe the city's demographics. The same data were researched for the state and nation for comparison purposes.

In July 2017, the students completed a windshield survey of the housing located in the city. Students, under the guidance of their faculty leads, developed an eight-question survey to be filled out to describe the housing in the city. The students, after delineating quadrants of the city to survey, divided up into teams and detailed the housing seen in each quadrant using the developed questionnaire.

In August 2017, a presentation was given to the staff of EPA, Region 5, to provide an update on the project. To assess the level of knowledge about radon among landlords with properties located in the city, a 23-question survey was developed by the research team. Landlords' knowledge of radon, along with willingness to test for radon and pay for mitigation, if needed, was assessed. A total of 92 surveys were distributed at two required landlord trainings held in October and November 2017. A response rate of 51% was achieved, with 47 surveys being completed.

The results of the survey showed that the majority of landlords had been renting properties for less than 1 year, owned one property, did not allow smoking in their properties, and rented for the purpose of additional income. Notably, 84.4% had not tested their rental properties for radon. The survey respondents also demonstrated a willingness to test for radon but needed more information about how to test, ways to mitigate their properties' exposure, and the costs for each.

The results of this survey were used to develop the ordinance proposal as well as the health communication campaign on radon.

Summary Points

1. The project took approximately 1 year to complete, during which time the team worked alongside community stakeholders with collaboration from local, state, and federal officials.
2. Landlords were receptive to radon testing within residential areas, but more education needed to be completed with both residents and landlords regarding the dangers of radon along with the consequences of long-term exposure to this gas.
3. The ordinance was drafted and submitted to local community public stakeholders for consideration and adoption.
4. Through the efforts of student, academic, and political stakeholders, it was possible to create further awareness regarding radon, the hazards of radon, and possible legislation at the local and state levels at the moment.

▶ Application of CEPH MPH Competencies

Many foundational competencies can be discussed regarding public health as well as work out in the field when performing research. Regarding this particular study, three areas can be identified regarding the foundational competencies: (1) evidence-based approaches to public health, (2) policy in public health, and (3) planning and management to promote health. The application of the research based on any information that was accrued during this particular study promised to have positive social change implications not only for the community but also for dealing with the landlords within the apartment complexes that were leasing and renting these particular units. This case study addresses CEPH competencies 9, 13, and 15.

Competency 9: Design a Population-Based Policy, Program, Project, or Intervention

For the purposes of this project, a quantitative approach was used to identify some of the key areas that were impacted by radon exposure. A windshield survey was completed in the early phases of the research. The results of this survey, which represented an observational method, served as the foundation for the remainder of the study. This particular project was conducted in Kane County, Illinois, in conjunction with the EPA Region 5 as well as local city officials. The purpose of this project was to examine which prevention initiatives could successfully promote awareness and educate landlords about radon, radon testing, and mitigation as well as to develop the various partnerships required for radon testing. To promote further education of the community regarding radon and radon testing, several stakeholders were identified during the course of the research: public agencies, nonprofit organizations, research institutions, and academia.

Further research demonstrated that about half of the Kane County homes and buildings tested between 2003 and 2011 demonstrated high levels of radon. Landlords were considered the largest group of stakeholders within the county. These landlords were divided into two groups: (1) landlords who did not inhabit the property and (2) landlords who were inhabiting the property. It was hypothesized that the landlords who were not inhabiting the properties would be more likely to resist testing for radon to keep their costs down. Conversely, it was hypothesized that the landlords who were also tenants, or inhabitants of the affected properties, would be more likely to test for radon, and would more willing to implement any mitigation strategies that might be available. It was determined that further evaluation and research studies regarding landlords, radon, and mitigation practices should be performed in an effort to understand completely the results.

Competency 13: Propose Strategies to Identify Stakeholders and Build Coalitions and Partnerships for Influencing Public Health Outcomes

This project revealed that there are minimal radon testing policies not only in the state of Illinois, but also throughout United States. To fully understand the economic impact of radon testing, mitigation strategies and policy development need to be implemented. Upon acquisition of the results of this study, a policy/ordinance was developed for the particular location covered by the study. This ordinance sought to create a foundation based on which political stakeholders, community representatives, and landlords would be able to work alongside one another in an effort to determine best practices for radon testing.[8,9] The proposed ordinance that was developed was the first of its kind for this particular county. Although the ordinance was drafted and then submitted, an overall strategy is still needed to make a positive social change and impact within that community.

The suggested public health policy pertaining to radon included a definition of terms, requirements for testing, mitigation strategies, and identification of violations. The researchers collaborated with county officials to replicate the template for the particular ordinance in an effort to perhaps "pass" the ordinance within the city council. Some of the key areas that were impactful regarding the draft ordinance pertained to 32 Illinois Administrative Code 422. In an effort to be compliant with this code, radon testing would need to be done on each property being released within 18 months from the effective date of the ordinance. It was also suggested that radon testing, if not performed within the context of the 32 Illinois Administrative Code 422, would not be accepted.

The team suggested that radon testing be completed every 5 years from the date of the last test. Further mitigation strategies were also included in the ordinance, including requirements for the tenant's notification of the result in writing from the landlord within 45 days of the test's completion. In essence, if the property being released has not yet had radon testing completed, the tenant must be notified in writing that testing has not been conducted within the given time frame. In regard to the violations, if the property is found not to have been tested, the owner/landlord could be fined as much as $1200 for each property. In addition, the testing would need to be done within 1 year of the violation.

Competency 15: Evaluate Policies for Their Impact on Public Health and Health Equity

In the research conducted for this particular project, there was a sincere attempt to assess the population needs, to look at the impact of the issue on the community's health, and to determine how the team could make a positive social change by creating an ordinance that would be beneficial for all parties involved. This ordinance would be applicable to all cultures. In addition, the team sought to implement a public health policy—in this case, through an ordinance, and perhaps by establishing programs that would benefit both tenants and landlords. The evaluation concluded there was a need for a population-based policy, some type of program development, or an intervention that would benefit tenants and landlords by clarifying the risks of radon. Some of the basic principles of the policy were making radon test kits available, but more importantly levying a heavy penalty on landlords who did not test for radon. Of course, money can never compensate for the value of a human life unnecessarily affected by cancer, but at least the economic losses might provide a stimulus for other states, and perhaps a federal mandate, to require testing for radon. It may take several attempts to pass state legislation regarding radon testing in duplexes, rental units, and apartment complexes, but the benefit to the inhabitants of those locations will be substantial—perhaps lowering some of the cancer rates that are associated with radon.

Discussion Questions

1. What are some of the locations within residential areas where radon can be found?
2. What were some of the initial findings related to radon exposure, and how did those findings affect future health and surveillance of health issues?
3. How will public health policy be impacted by performing radon research in residential settings?
4. Why is it important to have planning and management to promote public health and radon research?
5. Were the appropriate steps followed to draft the ordinance proposal? If not, list the correct steps that should be followed.

References

1. George, A. C. (2008). World history of radon research and measurement from the early 1900's to today. *AIP Conference Proceedings, 1034,* 20–33.
2. Bain, A. A., Abbott, A. L., & Miller, L. L. (2016). Successes and challenges in implementation of radon control activities in Iowa, 2010–2015. *Preventing Chronic Disease, 13,* E50. http://doi.org/10.5888/pcd13.150596
3. U.S. Environmental Protection Agency. (2013). *Consumer's guide to radon reduction: How to fix your home.* Retrieved from https://www.epa.gov/sites/production/files/2016-02/documents/2013_consumers_guide_to_radon_reduction.pdf
4. Wichmann, H. E., Rosario, A. S., Heid, I. M., Kreuzer, M., Heinrich, J., & Kreienbrock, L. (2005). Increased lung cancer risk due to residential radon in a pooled and extended analysis of studies in Germany. *Health Physics, 88*(1), 71–79.
5. Lougue, J. M., McKone, T. E., Sherman, M. H., & Singer, B. C. (2011). Hazard assessment measured in residence. *Indoor Air, 21*(2), 92–109.
6. Spengler, J. D., & Sexton, K. (1983). Indoor air pollution: A public health perspective. *Science, 221*(4605), 9–17.
7. Weinstein, N., Klotz, M., & Sandman, P. (1988). Optimistic biases in public perceptions of the risk from radon. *American Journal of Public Health, 78,* 796–800.
8. Hubaux, R., Becker-Santos, D. D., Enfield, K. S., Lam, S., Lam, W. L., & Martinez, V. D. (2012). Arsenic, asbestos and radon: Emerging players in lung tumorigenesis. *Environmental Health, 11,* 89.
9. Professional Radon Systems. (2014). Radon mitigation services. Retrieved from http://proradon.com/

CHAPTER 10

Ryan White HIV/AIDS Program Priority Setting and Resource Management Process

Anthony J. Santella, DrPH, MCHES

Georgette Beal, MHA

▶ Background

Human immunodeficiency virus (HIV)/acquired immunodeficiency syndrome (AIDS) and other sexually transmitted infections continue to be of public health significance in the United States. At the end of 2015, an estimated 1.1 million people older than the age of 13 were living with HIV in the United States. This includes approximately 162,000 people living with HIV/AIDS (PLWH/A) but unaware of their status. Despite advances in prevention methods and technologies, we continue to see a static number of new HIV diagnoses. In 2016, 39,782 people were newly diagnosed with HIV.[1]

Of the people who are aware of their HIV status, almost half (49%) are virally suppressed. Among people who have achieved viral suppression, HIV is detectable only at very low levels in the blood or is undetectable with standard tests. Viral suppression allows people with HIV to live longer, healthier lives and dramatically reduces their risk of transmitting HIV.[2]

The U.S. federal government's Ryan White HIV/AIDS Program, funded most recently by the Ryan White HIV/AIDS Treatment Extension Act of 2009, provides medical care and social support services to people living with HIV who are either uninsured or underinsured. The program is the largest federal government program designed to provide services to people living with HIV. It also serves as a payer of last resort to address the unmet care and treatment needs of people living with HIV/AIDS. The Ryan White program is managed by the Health Resources and Services Administration (HRSA) and funds programs in those cities most severely affected by the HIV epidemic (Part A); programs in states and territories to improve quality, availability, and organization of HIV services (Part B); community-based organizations at the local level to support early intervention services and ambulatory care (Part C); care and support for women, infant, and children living with HIV (Part D); and research, technical assistance, and access-to-care programs (Part F).[3]

The Part A grantees are legislatively required to have a Planning Council made up of appointed people living with HIV, medical and social services providers, researchers, and government officials, who are responsible for making decisions about service priorities and resource allocation. The Planning Council also assesses the service needs of people living with HIV in its geographic area, and the kinds and amount of services required to meet those needs. Moreover, it issues service directives to ensure high-quality and consistent services in the eligible metropolitan area (EMA). Members decide which services are most important to people living with HIV in the EMA (priority setting) and then agree on which service categories to fund and how much funding to provide (resource allocations).[4]

This case study focuses on the Nassau and Suffolk Counties, New York (e.g., Long Island) Planning Council's priority setting and resource allocation (PSRA) process.

▶ Case Study

The Nassau–Suffolk region utilizes a two-part collaborative process to set priorities and allocate resources for federal funding through Ryan White Part A. This PSRA process enables the Nassau–Suffolk EMA to identify regional HIV/AIDS priorities and to allocate funding to services that are most needed on Long Island. PSRA is highly data driven and incorporates many checks and balances to avoid conflicts of interest and ensure the best results. Priority setting brings all facets of the continuum of care (consumers, community stakeholders, and providers) to the table to examine data sources (surveys, public community forums, and needs assessments) with the goals of maximizing the provision of services to PLWH/A and ensuring resources go to the areas where services are most needed. Resource allocation entails an intensive review of epidemiologic data, program utilization data, other funding sources, and priority-setting outcomes to select priority funding amounts. PSRA is a vital tool that enables the EMA to meet its grant responsibilities as the payer of last resort.

In the Nassau–Suffolk region, PSRA is conducted by the Ryan White Part A Planning Council with participation of the Ryan White Part A Grantee, community-based providers, hospitals, consumers, and other community members. The Planning Council's Strategic Assessment and Planning (SAP) Committee is responsible for the priority-setting aspect of PSRA. SAP members who work at Ryan White Part A–funded agencies cannot vote on the priorities they represent but are able to actively participate in all discussions.

The Finance Subcommittee is responsible for resource allocation. Its membership consists of non-aligned consumers (those who do not work for or sit on boards of funded agencies), community leaders, and other individuals who are unaffiliated with agencies that are recipients of Ryan White Part A funds. As part of the checks and balances system, the SAP Committee receives recommendations from the Finance Subcommittee for approval; a full report is then presented to the Planning Council for final vote and approval. Committee and Planning Council members whose agencies are funded by Part A cannot vote on the priorities they represent but are able to actively participate in all discussions.

Prior to commencing the PSRA process, a work plan is developed to outline committee responsibilities and to guide decision making. The work plan describes the agreed-upon methodology, criteria, procedures, and desired outcome; confirms program mandates; and directs the gathering of the latest data and information/inputs. Data for priority setting include information gathered during annual community forums, through consumer and provider surveys, and from periodic needs assessments conducted on special populations. A dedicated data review session is conducted for both the SAP Committee and Finance Subcommittee to examine quantitative and qualitative data on barriers, gaps, needs, and costs. Particular attention is paid to data that highlight barriers to care access for minority populations when selecting and allocating funding.

Priority Setting

The PSRA process commences with the SAP Committee reviewing and analyzing available data sources (**TABLE 10-1**), with its goal being to gain a better understanding of the impact of the HIV/AIDS epidemic in the EMA. The SAP Committee sets priorities using a predetermined agenda that incorporates member disclosure of conflicts of interest, review of principles and criteria, listing of services as allowable under the Ryan White program, review of the previous year's priorities, the goals and objectives from the most recent Integrated HIV Prevention and Care Plan, the National HIV/AIDS Monitoring Standards, Health Resources and Services Administration (HRSA) mandates on the use of funds, and an epidemiology/surveillance data presentation. The data are thoroughly examined and revisions are made when sufficient and compelling evidence warrants a change.

Upon review and discussion, the SAP Committee selects from a list of 28 HRSA-allowable services. From this list, the committee ranks services deemed the most important and most needed by PLWH/A in care. Ranked priorities include those with the overall goal of improving viral load suppression as well as those most critical to addressing goals in the New York State Integrated HIV Prevention and Care Plan and Ending the Epidemic Blueprint. The remaining services are ranked as needed for PLWH/A but not recommended for allocation due to coverage in the region from other funding sources, such as local programs, state programs, Medicaid, Medicare, the Centers for Disease Control and Prevention, and the Substance Abuse and Mental Health Services Administration. A written report with the ranked priority list and rationale is sent to the Finance Subcommittee for use in resource allocation.

TABLE 10-1 Sample Data and Process for the Priority-Setting Process

Data Reviewed	Link to Plan Goals	Recommend
▪ Updated epidemiologic data ▪ Consumer survey results ▪ Community meetings results ▪ Provider survey results ▪ "Out of care" needs assessment ▪ "In care" needs assessments for African American/Black, Hispanic, women of color, men having sex with men (MSM), and individuals age 45 and older ▪ Unmet need framework (diagnosed HIV but not in care) ▪ Cascade of care for Nassau–Suffolk Counties ▪ Goals and objectives from New York State Integrated HIV Prevention and Care Plan ▪ Health Resources and Services Administration–defined list of Part A–fundable service priorities	▪ SAP Committee "links" priorities for the next fiscal years to goals as outlined in the eligible metropolitan area's most recent Integrated HIV Prevention and Care Plan	▪ Strategic Assessment and Planning (SAP) Committee priority list with rankings and recommendations goes to the Finance Subcommittee ▪ Finance Subcommittee recommendations and allocation chart go back to the SAP Committee ▪ Final recommendation is made to Planning Council on service priorities and resource allocations

Source: Data from Planning and Grants Management Department, United Way of Long Island, May 2018.

Resource Allocation

The Finance Subcommittee meets approximately 1 week after the SAP Committee and also follows the process outlined in the work plan to make its allocation recommendations. An Excel spreadsheet is prepared for the committee that includes six charts designed to assist the committee in determining how much Ryan White Part A funding is needed to support the comprehensive system of HIV/AIDS care on Long Island. The charts offer a mechanism for members to compare previous award levels; evaluate data on the current number of HIV-positive individuals being served by Ryan White Part A; review data on newly diagnosed persons as well as previously diagnosed individuals who are out of care; and estimate the costs to maintain individuals who are currently being served in addition to bringing new individuals into the service system.

The Finance Subcommittee reviews data such as those listed in **TABLE 10-2** to assist in determining the needs of individuals who HIV positive but are not in care, those who are unaware of their status, and those who are historically underserved.

The committee begins its deliberations by examining the total amount available to the Nassau–Suffolk EMA based on the cap HRSA sets for each EMA as part of its annual grant application process. As of 2017, EMAs and Transitional Grant Areas (TGAs) may request no more than 5% of the previous year's level funding

TABLE 10-2 Data and Process Used in Resource Allocation Process		
Data Sets Reviewed by Finance Subcommitee	**Resource Allocation Components**	**Resource Allocation Percentages**
Unduplicated clients by units of service and by unit cost per client	1: Current clients receiving Ryan White Part A or Minority AIDS Initiative (MAI) services.	Resource allocation percentages are developed and approved by the Planning Council based on the total grant request.
Most recent epidemiologic data available	2: The expected number of new clients based on the eligible metropolitan area's Epidemiological Profile (the committee sets a percentage of the total).	These percentages will be applied to the service dollars upon the notice of grant award.
Most recent unmet needs framework	3: Estimated number needing but not receiving services and the additional cost to serve these clients.	
Other funding sources by service category	4: A goal is set by the Finance Subcommittee to bring a percentage of the unaware individuals into care. Additional funds are allocated for each service priority for this population.	

amount. With that in mind, the committee looks at the number of clients who are currently being served in the Ryan White Part A service system and sets an additional goal to bring a certain percentage of newly diagnosed and unaware individuals into care. The current cost per client for each funded priority is applied to these numbers and used to estimate the number and costs for clients to be served in 2019. If this formula results in a total grant ask amount that exceeds the 5% cap, then the committee uses expenditure data as well as information about other public funding to decrease the amounts allocated to certain priorities by reducing the projected number of clients to be served. Once the budget is balanced and the committee is satisfied with the allocations, motions are made and votes on taken on allocations for each priority individually.

Based on the Finance Subcommittee's recommendation to the SAP Committee and a final vote by SAP, a recommendation is presented to the full Planning Council for a vote. The council votes on the rankings, amounts, and percentages by priority and on a total grant "ask" amount. If the final award amount provided by HRSA differs from the grant ask amount, the council uses the percentages that were voted on for each priority to reallocate funds.

Summary Points

1.   A well-articulated budget and resource allocation/management process is needed to ensure transparency and active participation by all stakeholders.
2.   When undergoing a budget and resource allocation/management process with both public health professionals and community members, sufficient time should be allocated for reviewing, explaining, and interpreting budget principles and for interpreting the data used to make decisions.
3.   The use of data from multiple sources is key to making sound resource allocation decisions for supporting decisions to increase or decrease funds to budget lines.

▶ Application of CEPH MPH Competencies

This case study addresses CEPH competencies 10 and 17.

Competency 10: Explain Basic Principles and Tools of Budget and Resource Management

The Planning Council administrative staff, who are employed by the United Way of Long Island, are tasked with leading this effort, along with the co-chairs of the SAP Committee. Due to the turnover of SAP Committee members each year, PSRA content and process training is repeated on an annual basis before the PSRA process begins. This process includes principles of budget management so that committee members understand not only the budgeting process but also the costs associated with providing each of the HRSA-approved services. Additional topics covered in the training include the legislative requirements associated with receiving Ryan White federal funding and how changes in healthcare financing impact the PSRA process. Although the training takes place in just one session, questions are answered during each session to ensure each committee member is comfortable making budget decisions.

With respect to the resource management process, the Planning Council must approve any reallocation of funds among service categories. This type of reallocation usually means moving funds to other providers within the same service category or to service categories who are exceeding their spending goals and have additional need. Expenditure data are reviewed periodically to facilitate this process.

Competency 17: Apply Negotiation and Mediation Skills to Address Organizational or Community Challenges

As one could imagine, getting both the SAP Committee and the full Planning Council to approve one priority setting and resource allocation plan can be challenging. Sometimes conflicts arise, for reasons such as fear of defunding services, need to support organizational versus individual priorities and challenges, and lack of understanding of the population-level epidemiology and surveillance data, among other things. Despite these limitations, the SAP Committee and Planning Council are always able to achieve a consensus vote on each of the funded services that are being requested to HRSA. When conflict has emerged between SAP and/or Planning Council members, a number of techniques have been used to mediate the situation: review of the process/data used to arrive at decisions, gathering of additional data on areas of concern/question, and allowing individuals involved in conflict to voice their concern and goals. Moreover, the Planning Council staff and chairs ensure that all Planning Council members are able to examine resource allocation scenarios from the perspectives of others and to identify areas of agreement among their diverse membership. Where the SAP Committee and the Planning Council cannot come to an agreement, the council has a final vote.

Discussion Questions

1. What strengths and weaknesses can you identify for the budget and resource allocation/management process done by the Nassau–Suffolk Ryan White Planning Council? How would you change the weaknesses?
2. If you were the chair of the SAP Committee or chair of the Planning Council, what steps would you take to ensure all members (ranging from consumers without formal education to physicians and other providers) understand the basic budget principles and resource allocation/management processes?
3. How would you manage the conflicts of interest that arise when providers and consumers try to influence a vote on allocations to meet their own needs?

References

1. Centers for Disease Control and Prevention. (2018, June 26). HIV surveillance report. Retrieved from https://www.cdc.gov/hiv/statistics/overview/index.html
2. Centers for Disease Control and Prevention. (2017, July 27). More people with HIV have the virus under control. Retrieved from https://www.cdc.gov/nchhstp/newsroom/2017/2017-HIV-Continuum-Press-Release.html
3. Health Resources and Services Administration. (2016, October). About the Ryan White HIV/AIDS program. Retrieved from https://hab.hrsa.gov/about-ryan-white-hivaids-program/about-ryan-white-hivaids-program
4. Ryan White HIV/AIDS Program. (2018, June). *Planning Council primer.* Retrieved from https://careacttarget.org/sites/default/files/file-upload/resources/Primer_June2018.pdf

CHAPTER 11

Evaluating a Multi-Site Campus-Based Sexual Assault Prevention Intervention

Spring Chenoa Cooper, PhD
Claudia Wald, MSW

▶ Background

Facing new scrutiny by the federal government, adjudicators, and media, colleges throughout the United States have been reevaluating their approaches to campus sexual assault.[1,2] College-age women in the United States have been experiencing elevated, yet still under-reported, rates of sexual assault and intimate-partner violence (IPV) for several decades.[3–5] IPV involves physical violence, sexual violence, stalking, and psychological aggression (including coercive acts) by a current or former intimate partner.[6] It is important to have a uniform definition of IPV to ensure that public health surveillance system information is collected in a systematic fashion for the health outcome under surveillance. It has been repeatedly reported that one in five college women experiences sexual assault or attempted sexual assault.[4,7,8] This is a notoriously under-reported crime, however, so real rates are likely to be even higher.[8,9] In almost 80% of sexual violence incidents among 18- to 24-year-olds, the survivor knew the perpetrator, indicating that the majority of college-age sexual assault involves either IPV or acquaintance sexual assault.[9]

The high occurrence of sexual violence on college campuses is problematic for many reasons, including the threats it poses to students' physical, emotional, mental, and sexual health, which in turn impacts their academic and lifetime achievements.[9,10,11–16] The aftermath of IPV and sexual violence can affect survivors' physical, social, financial, and emotional well-being.[17,18] Victimized women are far more likely to experience more disabling and life-threatening consequences of abuse,[11,19,20] whose effects often extend throughout their lifetime and put them at risk for repeat victimization.[21]

The City University of New York (CUNY) is a large, urban, commuter college. The university is composed of 24 institutions in New York City, with a student body of more than half a million people (269,000 degree-credit students and 247,000 adult, continuing education, and professional education students). CUNY includes 11 senior colleges, 7 community colleges, the Macaulay Honors College, and 5 graduate and professional schools, located throughout the city's five boroughs. In the fall semester of 2016, CUNY undergraduates were 32% Hispanic, 26% Black, 21% White, and 21% Asian/Pacific Islander.[22] CUNY is made up of underserved populations: in 2016, 37% were foreign-born, 42% had annual household incomes less than $20,000, 45% were the first generation in their families to attend college, and 27% worked more than 20 hours per week.[22]

Despite CUNY's efforts to propel low-socioeconomic-status students into higher levels, a great majority of students do not complete their degrees: Only 53% of CUNY's students in baccalaureate or associate degree programs complete their degree within 10 years of enrollment, and many never finish because of health issues. This could be related to the fact that commuter colleges are often unable to deliver health and preventive services to all or most students when compared to residential colleges' ability to do so.[11,23] Overall, only a scant 13% of beginning college students live on the CUNY campus, with approximately 50% commuting and 33% living with parents or family—facts that make it all the more urgent to modernize our conception of the "traditional" college student.[24] Commuter students commute for reasons of age, lifestyle, family circumstances, and financial need. Additionally, many of the minority students enrolled at CUNY come from ethnic backgrounds that place a strong emphasis on the preservation of the family unit. In a recent study at the City College of New York, the flagship campus of CUNY, four health domains were identified as being consistently linked to academic problems: mental health, sexual and reproductive health, healthcare access, and hunger and food insecurity. In examining the sexual and reproductive health domain, researchers found that sexual assault and IPV are pervasive issues for CUNY students.[11]

Most sexual violence prevention strategies in the evaluation literature are short-term programs focused on increasing knowledge or changing attitudes, which have not shown to be effective when subjected to rigorous evaluation.[25] Only three primary prevention strategies have demonstrated significant effects on sexually violent behavior in a rigorous outcome evaluation, which could be adapted for use in university settings: Safe Dates,[26] Shifting Boundaries (building-level intervention only),[27] and funding associated with the 1994 U.S. Violence Against Women Act. With the majority of college students in the United States attending commuter schools,[24] there is a need for prevention programming to be grounded in data that come from such institutions.

▶ Case Study

Sexual assault and IPV are pressing problems to combat among college students, for which monitoring and evaluation of student safety measures is critically needed. Rather than focusing on nationally representative population-level data, it behooves scholars to focus on collecting nuanced data that can provide more typologies of colleges and college students in terms of commuter student populations.[11] Data that help us understand different populations of commuter students are rare, however. If such data were more accessible, we could create more meaningful analyses of sexual assault and IPV risk for commuter students and tailor interventions to those populations.

Intervention Description

This intervention is aligned with recent scholarship focusing on primary prevention of sexual assault—which is seen as the most cost-effective approach and one that is beneficial to community welfare—and thereby expanding the evidence base beyond secondary and tertiary prevention approaches (e.g., treatment or recidivism prevention), strategies targeting victimization prevention (i.e., risk reduction), or research on the etiology of sexual assault.[25] Sexual agency is defined as the ability by young people to take "control of who can take sexual pleasure from their bodies … [as] They learn to take responsibility for making their own decisions."[28] For young people, taking agency means that they do not simply do what parents, teachers, or friends tell them, but instead make informed and ethical choices for themselves and accept the responsibility of those choices. A community with a high level of sexual agency may have lower rates of sexual assault.

The Healthy Relationships Intervention, developed by the research team in concert with established CUNY-wide activities, aims to improve a community level of sexual agency through various means by targeting students at different ecological levels.

Safe and Healthy Relationships Focus Groups and Intervention Development

The research team, led by the authors of this chapter, conducted focus groups at the seven CUNY campuses, collecting information about and perceptions of the ways that sexual and relationship violence is addressed by each school. These data, coupled with exhaustive research on best practices to prevent college-wide sexual assault, informed the development of the Healthy Relationships Intervention to be implemented at CUNY schools.

The social–ecological framework is a multifaceted conceptual framework to study violence: this framework applies various ecologies to understand complex behaviors such as violence.[25] The Healthy Relationships Intervention, developed by the research team in concert with established CUNY-wide activities, aims to foster a higher level of sexual agency across the community through various means by targeting students at different ecological levels.

Planned interventions target different ecological levels (**TABLE 11-1**), including opt-in texting (direct links to information and reminders; users may text questions back) at the individual level; consent trainings for students (peer-led; sustainable over several years) at the peer level; social norming and branding through posters; agency trainings—knowledge/skills missing from consent/bystander, including negotiation, gender/culture examinations, practicing communication, and bystander trainings for students and faculty/staff; and, at the

TABLE 11-1 Goals of Intervention and Outcomes		
Goals	**Tasks**	**Outcomes**
Students demonstrate an understanding of the complexities surrounding consent; demonstrate the ability to recognize a potentially dangerous situation, know how to intervene, and are able to take active steps toward intervention; and understand how to best support peers who have experienced sexual assault.	■ Implement agency and consent trainings ■ Implement bystander trainings ■ Implement branding activities ■ Develop and disseminate continuing education videos online	Students receive factual information about sexuality, communication, sexual assault, and recovery.
Survivors have access to quality care, 24 hours a day, 7 days a week, facilitated through CUNY.	■ Ensure that survivors receive an advocate ■ Advocate follows up to assist in referral process	Survivors feel supported and have accessed appropriate services.
CUNY campuses will not tolerate sexual victimization; the CUNY culture is one of acceptance.	■ Implement large social norming campaign ■ Implement educational materials ■ Engage underserved populations	Reduced incidence of sexual assault.
CUNY campuses will take active steps toward creating a campus of support.	■ Implement large social norming campaign ■ Implement all of the educational materials	Reduced stigma around communication about sexuality, LGBTQ issues, and sexual assault survivors.

CUNY level, implementation of social norming and branding through social media and websites.

At the societal level, the ecological approach of a coordinated community response approach provides for the development of campus-wide responses involving campus victim service providers, law enforcement/campus safety officers, health providers, housing officials, administrators, student leaders, faith-based leaders, and representatives from student organizations and connections to local off-campus criminal justice agencies and service providers, including local law enforcement agencies, prosecutors' offices, courts, and nonprofit, nongovernmental victim advocacy and victim services organizations.

Summary Points

1. The new multilevel approach to campus sexual assault prevention programming uses primary prevention methods.
2. Complex intervention design: The most successful interventions are those that are complex and cross several ecological levels.
3. The case study is an example of academic researchers working within their university system to effect change related to a public health issue.
4. Outcome measures are tied directly back to the goals of the intervention.

▶ Application of CEPH MPH Competencies

This case study addresses CEPH competencies 11 and 2.

Competency 11: Select Methods to Evaluate Public Health Programs

Each intervention activity is matched to an evaluation measure that will assess how the intervention activity is related to the intervention goals and outcomes (**TABLE 11-2**). In choosing methods to evaluate the intervention activities, existing data are considered first, to minimize both cost and workload. Where appropriate existing data are not available, measures are implemented to assess the intervention component.

We have chosen pre- and post-surveys to demonstrate changes in measured outcomes and to show that the intervention is the causal agent in these shifts. Additionally, random samples are proposed for campus-wide or university-wide initiatives so that we can maximize the generalizability of our results.

TABLE 11-2 Intervention Components		
Ecological Model Level	**Intervention Activity**	**Evaluation Measure**
Individual level	Online training (already happening; CUNY-wide implemented initiative)	Existing data we can utilize: Online training completion rates
Small group/ friends level	Clubs at individual campuses in creating events around intervention themes Request-a-Party (opt-in safer sex parties)	Rates of club involvement Pre-/post-surveys with students who engage with safer sex educational parties
Family level	Process for students to invite family members to agency trainings with them	Qualitative feedback with family members who wish to participate

(continues)

TABLE 11-2	Intervention Components	*(continued)*
Campus level	*Agency trainings* (includes consent) *Bystander trainings* for students and faculty/staff Radio spots on campuses that have stations Safe spaces at each campus for LGBTQ and victim support Social norming and branding through posters Branding materials given at freshmen orientations and through wellness centers	Pre-/post-surveys with students who attend trainings Pre-/post-random-sample of campus students measuring: ■ Sociodemographics ■ Knowledge of agency training ■ Knowledge of consent training ■ Knowledge of bystander training ■ Attitudes about masculinity ■ Negotiation and communication skills self-efficacy ■ Behaviors Qualitative focus groups with students Existing data we can utilize: ■ CUNY Campus Climate Surveys ■ Academic achievement rates ■ CUNY sexual assault data
CUNY-wide level	Social norming and branding through social media and websites Videos demonstrating and showing how to practice different skills (7–8 over each semester) Online advice columns to which students can submit questions Contests (for prizes) where students create materials, in any media, for wider circulation	Random sample pre-/post-survey of CUNY students measuring awareness of the campaign Social media statistics Existing data we can utilize: ■ Healthy CUNY surveys on health outcomes ■ Police sexual assault data

Competency 2: Select Quantitative and Qualitative Data Collection Methods Appropriate for a Given Public Health Context

Choosing evaluation procedures and techniques for the intervention is as important as designing the intervention. If we do not choose the correct methods and measures for evaluation, we cannot be sure that our intervention is having the desired effects. In some instances, we will use validated measures that will give us indications of how much an indicator of interest has shifted; in other instances, we will create our own measures to meet our specific needs. In addition, we have chosen to apply a qualitative methodology (focus groups) that will give us a more exploratory option to investigate both the effects and potential confounders we may not have anticipated.

Discussion Questions

1. Why would it be important to address summative evaluation (the degree to which actual changes occurred as a result of the program) as opposed to limiting assessment to process evaluation?
2. What types of outcomes might have more value in health promotion, as well as in reducing the burden of sexual assault and intimate-partner violence, in a large, urban, commuter university setting?
3. Why might policy-makers and funders be more concerned with summative evaluation outcomes than with process-based outcomes?

References

1. It's On Us. (n.d.). Homepage. Retrieved from http://www.itsonus.org/
2. Remarks by the president at "It's On Us" campaign rollout. (2014, September 19). Retrieved from https://obamawhitehouse.archives.gov/the-press-office/2014/09/19/remarks-president-its-us-campaign-rollout
3. Muehlenhard, C. L., Peterson, Z. D., Humphreys, T. P., & Jozkowski, K. N. (2017). Evaluating the one-in-five statistic: Women's risk of sexual assault while in college. *Journal of Sex Research, 54*(4–5), 549–576. doi:10.1080/00224499.2017.1295014
4. Fisher, B. S., Cullen, F. T., & Turner, M. G. (2000, December). The sexual victimization of college women: Research report. Retrieved from https://eric.ed.gov/?id=ED449712
5. Krebs, C., Lindquist, C., Warner, T., Fisher, B., & Martin, S. (2007). *The Campus Sexual Assault (CSA) study*. Washington, DC: U.S. Department of Justice. Retrieved from https://www.ncjrs.gov/pdffiles1/nij/grants/221153.pdf
6. Black, M. C., Basile, K. C., Breiding, M. J., Smith, S. G., Walters, M. L., Merrick, M. T., ... & Stevens, M. R. (2011). *The National Intimate Partner and Sexual Violence Survey (NISVS): 2010 summary report*. Atlanta, GA: National Center for Injury Prevention and Control, Centers for Disease Control and Prevention. Retrieved from https://www.cdc.gov/violenceprevention/pdf/nisvs_executive_summary-a.pdf
7. Sinozich, S., & Langton, L. (2014). *Rape and sexual assault victimization among college-age females, 1995–2013*. Washington, DC: U.S. Department of Justice, Office of Justice Programs, Bureau of Justice Statistics. Retrieved from https://www.bjs.gov/content/pub/pdf/rsavcaf9513.pdf
8. Cantor, D., Fisher, B., Chibnall, S., Bruce, C., Townsend, R., Thomas, G., & Lee, H. (2015, September 21). *Report on the AAU Campus Climate Survey on Sexual Assault and Sexual Misconduct*. Charlottesville, VA: University of Virginia. Retrieved from https://assets.documentcloud.org/documents/2674806/University-of-Virginia-Climate-Survey.pdf
9. 2011 college dating violence and abuse poll. (2011, June 9). Retrieved from http://www.loveisrespect.org/pdf/College_Dating_And_Abuse_Final_Study.pdf
10. Tsui, E. K., & Santamaria, E. K. (2015). Intimate partner violence risk among undergraduate women from an urban commuter college: The role of navigating off- and on-campus social environments. *Journal of Urban Health, 92*(3), 513–526. doi:10.1007/s11524-014-9933-0
11. Centers for Disease Control and Prevention, Injury Center. (2018, October 23). Violence prevention: Definitions: Intimate partner violence. Retrieved from https://www.cdc.gov/violenceprevention/intimatepartnerviolence/definitions.html

12. Flake, D. F. (2016, June). Individual, family, and community risk markers for domestic violence in Peru. *Violence Against Women*. doi:10.1177/1077801204272129

13. Bachar, K., & Koss, M. (2001). From prevalence to prevention: Closing the gap between what we know about rape and what we do. In C. M. Renzetti, J. L. Edleson, & R. K. Bergen (Eds.), *Sourcebook on violence against women* (pp. 117–142). London, UK: Sage Publications.

14. Campbell, R. (2013). The psychological impact of rape victims' experiences with the legal, medical, and mental health systems. In D. A. Sisti, A. L. Caplan, & H. Rimon-Greenspan (Eds.), *Applied ethics in mental health care: An interdisciplinary reader* (pp. 149–178). Cambridge, MA: MIT Press.

15. Jordan, C. E., Campbell, R., & Follingstad, D. (2010, March 24). Violence and women's mental health: The impact of physical, sexual, and psychological aggression. *Annual Review of Clinical Psychology, 6*, 607–628. doi: 10.1146/annurev-clinpsy-090209-151437

16. Halstead, V., Williams, J. R., & Gonzalez-Guarda, R. (2017, March). Sexual violence in the college population: A systematic review of disclosure and campus resources and services. *Journal of Clinical Nursing, 26*(15–16). doi:10.1111/jocn.13735

17. National Coalition Against Domestic Violence. (n.d.). Domestic Violence [Fact Sheet]. Retrieved from https://www.speakcdn.com/assets/2497/domestic_violence2.pdf

18. Federal Bureau of Investigation. (2012). Expanded homicide data: Table 10. Retrieved from https://ucr.fbi.gov/crime-in-the-u.s/2012/crime-in-the-u.s.-2012/offenses-known-to-law-enforcement/expanded-homicide/expanded_homicide_data_table_10_murder_circumstances_by_relationship_2012.xls

19. Daigle, L. E., Fisher, B. S., & Cullen, F. T. (2008). The violent and sexual victimization of college women: Is repeat victimization a problem? *Journal of Interpersonal Violence, 23*(9), 1296–1313. doi:10.1177/0886260508314293

20. Stayton, C., Olson, C., Thorpe, L., Kerker, B., Henning, K., & Wilt, S. (2008). *Intimate partner violence against women in New York City*. New York, NY: New York City Department of Health and Mental Hygiene. Retrieved from https://www1.nyc.gov/assets/doh/downloads/pdf/public/ipv-08.pdf

21. Kuh, G. D., Gonyea, R. M., & Palmer, M. (2001). *The disengaged commuter student: Fact or fiction?* Bloomington, IN: Indiana University Center for Postsecondary Research and Planning. Retrieved from http://nsse.indiana.edu/pdf/commuter.pdf

22. CUNY Office of Institutional Research and Assessment. (2015). Undergraduate Enrollment by Race/Ethnicity, Gender and College: Fall 2014 [Fact Sheet]. Retrieved from http://www.cuny.edu/irdatabook/rpts3_AY_archive/AY2014/ENRL_0032_RACE_GEN_UG.rpt.pdf

23. Frye, V., Galea, S., Tracy, M., Bucciarelli, A., Putnam, S., & Wilt, S. (2008). The role of neighborhood environment and risk of intimate partner femicide in a large urban area. *American Journal of Public Health, 98*(8), 1473–1479. doi:10.2105/AJPH.2007.112813

24. Deil-Amen, R. (2011). The "traditional" college student: A smaller and smaller minority and its implications for diversity and access institutions. *Mapping Broad-Access Higher Education Conference at Stanford University, 1*, 2014. Retrieved from https://cepa.stanford.edu/sites/default/files/2011%20Deil-Amen%2011_11_11.pdf

25. DeGue, S., Valle, L. A., Holt, M. K., Massetti, G. M., Matjasko, J. L., & Tharp, A. T. (2014). A systematic review of primary prevention strategies for sexual violence perpetration. *Aggressive and Violent Behavior, 19*(4), 346–362. doi:10.1016/j.avb.2014.05.004

26. Foshee, V. A., Bauman, K. E., Ennett, S. T., Linder, G. F., Benefield, T., & Suchindran, C. (2004). Assessing the long term effects of the Safe Dates program and a booster in preventing and reducing adolescent dating violence victimization and perpetration. *American Journal of Public Health, 94*(4), 619–624.

27. Taylor, B., Stein, N. D., Woods, D., & Mumford, E. (2011). *Shifting boundaries: Final report on an experimental evaluation of a youth dating violence prevention program in New York City middle schools (NCJ No. 236175)*. Rockville, MD: National Criminal Justice Reference Service (NCJRS). Retrieved from http://www.ncjrs.gov/App/publications/abstract.aspx?ID=258169

28. McKee, A., Albury, K., Dunne, M., Grieshaber, S., Hartley, J., Lumby, C., & Mathews, B. (2010). Healthy sexual development: A multidisciplinary framework for research. *International Journal of Sexual Health, 22*(1), 14–19.

Policy in Public Health

CHAPTER 12

Developing Primary Laws and Secondary Regulations for Food Safety: The Case of FSMA and Its Attendant Rules

Jason M. Ackleson, PhD
Sara E. Gragg, PhD
Justin J. Kastner, PhD
Ellyn R. Mulcahy, PhD, MPH
Daniel A. Unruh, PhD

▶ Background

The first major U.S. federal laws relating to food safety were the 1906 Pure Food and Drug Act and the 1907 Federal Meat Inspection Act.[1] Both laws won the support of Congress on the strength of the evidence for their need and ethical concerns (amplified by Upton Sinclair's *The Jungle*, which shed light on the poor sanitation practices in the Chicago meatpacking industry).[2] To tighten regulatory oversight of food safety for non-meat products, Congress passed the 1938 Federal Food Drug and Cosmetic Act, which superseded the Pure Food and Drug Act. Together, these laws, the 1957 Poultry Products Inspection Act, and the 1970 Egg Products Inspection Act formed the food safety foundation in the United States for many decades. In addition, the last century witnessed occasional congressional legislative action as well as frequent executive-level departmental rule-making related to food safety. These two levels (i.e., legislative and regulatory) of policy-making have routinely taken action on the basis of data collected, ethical values, public sentiment, and risk awareness. For example, following the terrorist attacks of September 11, 2001, and out of concerns about the vulnerability of the food system itself, Congress passed the 2002 Public Health Security and Bioterrorism Preparedness and Response Act, with executive departments (notably, the Food and Drug Administration [FDA]) adopting security regulations aimed at food imports.[1]

The major U.S. food safety laws mentioned previously remain important and are still codified at 21 United States Code (U.S.C.) § 301 et seq., 21 U.S.C. § 601 et seq., 21 U.S.C. § 451 et seq., and 21 U.S.C. § 1031 et seq., respectively. However, in the twenty-first century a new law was needed following ever-increasing foodborne illness outbreaks caused by virulent pathogens in numerous food vehicles in the 1990s and 2000s. This case study explores how evidence (acquired via the U.S. government's disease surveillance apparatus), ethics (nested in litigious liability precedents), and actors at different levels propelled Congress to pass, and the president to sign, a new law expanding FDA's enforcement powers: the 2011 FDA Food Safety Modernization Act (FSMA).

▶ Case Study

The Centers for Disease Control and Prevention (CDC), working alongside the FDA and the U.S. Department of Agriculture (USDA), conducts microbial surveillance—the tracking of foodborne illness through collection and analysis of data—to understand the quantity of and responsible microorganisms causing foodborne outbreaks in the United States. The CDC integrates data from state and local health agencies to achieve this goal. CDC-related programs track physician-reported outbreaks, molecular and genetic profiles of pathogens, and antimicrobial resistance patterns.[3,4] Principal among these programs are the Foodborne Disease Active Surveillance Network (FoodNet) and the National Molecular Subtyping Network for Foodborne Disease Surveillance. FoodNet interprets data from clinical laboratories to track infection diagnoses of several foodborne pathogens, including *Salmonella, Listeria,* and *Escherichia coli*.[5] PulseNet, a network of 83 laboratories, identifies foodborne illness outbreaks by comparing pulsed-field gel electrophoresis (PFGE) DNA fingerprints; this network results in quicker identification of illnesses and detection of outbreaks on a national scale.[6] Through the CDC's work, a number of pathogens have been identified as worrisome from a food safety perspective. These include bacterial and viral agents (as well as parasites) that are responsible for a significant number of illnesses, hospitalizations, and deaths (**TABLE 12-1**).[7,8]

Included in Table 12-1 is *Salmonella*, one of the bacteria most commonly (and historically) associated with foodborne infection. In 1994, *Salmonella* (in ice cream) was implicated in a widespread foodborne illness outbreak, catching the attention of policy-makers.[9] While not responsible for the same magnitude of illnesses, hospitalizations, and deaths as *Salmonella*, another genera of pathogens—Shiga toxin–producing *Escherichia coli* (STEC)—caught policy-makers' attention around the same time. In 1993, an outbreak of *E. coli* O157:H7 infection caused by consumption of hamburgers sold by the Jack-in-the-Box restaurant chain fueled alarm and anxiety, prompting the declaration of this organism as an adulterant in beef products and the eventual (in 1996) adoption of a new *E. coli* prevention-oriented regulation by the USDA's Food Safety and Inspection Service.[10,11] Over the next decade, a host of non-meat-related outbreaks confirmed that concerns about STEC (and *Salmonella*)

TABLE 12-1 Estimated Contributions of Various Pathogens to Illnesses, Hospitalizations, and Deaths Related to Foodborne Illness in the United States

Rank	Illnesses		Hospitalizations		Deaths	
	Pathogen	Number	Pathogen	Number	Pathogen	Number
1	Norovirus	5,461,731	Salmonella, nontyphoidal	19,336	Salmonella, nontyphoidal	378
2	Salmonella, nontyphoidal	1,027,561	Norovirus	14,633	Toxoplasma gondii	327
3	Clostridium perfringens	965,958	Campylobacter spp.	8,463	Listeria monocytogenes	255
4	Campylobacter spp.	845,024	Toxoplasma gondii	4,428	Norovirus	149
5	Staphylococcus aureus	241,148	E. coli (STEC) O157	2,138	Campylobacter spp.	76

Data from: Scallan, E., Hoekstra, R. M., Angulo, F. J., Tauxe, R. V., Widdowson, M.-A., Roy, S. L., . . . Griffin, P. M. (2011). Foodborne illness acquired in the United States—Major pathogens. *Emerging Infectious Diseases, 17*(1), 7–15. doi:10.3201/eid1701.P11101; Centers for Disease Control and Prevention. (2016). Burden of foodborne illness: Findings. Retrieved from https://www.cdc.gov/foodborneburden/index.html

transcended the meat industry and demanded a wider regulatory response; outbreaks of STEC infection caused by contamination of spinach (2006) and *Salmonella* infection caused by peppers (2008) and peanut butter (2009) begged questions about the FDA's regulatory powers and food companies' due diligence in food safety matters.[12,13] In the following years, several class-action lawsuits were filed against firms that produced or processed these contaminated foods; significantly, liability was attached to firms deemed to have been negligent, unethical, or both.[14]

The infectious dose of STEC, including but not limited to *E. coli* O157:H7, is as low as 10 cells, and the resultant disease can be particularly severe: bloody diarrhea, kidney failure, and, in some cases, death.[15–17] These concerning sequelae had already captured the attention of politicians across the country through the work of activist groups such as Safe Tables Our Priority (STOP) and groups such as the Center for Science in the Public Interest (CSPI). **TABLE 12-2** demonstrates how STEC, once thought to be solely responsible for outbreaks in beef (a USDA-regulated product),

TABLE 12-2 Selected Shiga Toxin–Producing *Escherichia coli* Outbreaks, 2008–2011

Year	Product	Strain	Cases (Hospitalizations, Deaths)
2008	Ground beef	O157:H7	49 (27, 0)
2009	Prepackaged cookie dough	O157:H7	72 (34, 0)
2009	Beef products	O157:H7	23 (12, 0)
2009	Ground beef	O157:H7	26 (19, 2)
2010	Ground beef	O157:H7	21 (9, 0)
2010	Shredded romaine lettuce	O145	30 (12, 0)
2010	Cheese	O157:H7	38 (15, 0)
2011	In-shell hazelnuts	O157:H7	8 (4, 0)
2011	Lebanon bologna	O157:H7	14 (3, 0)
2011	Travel to Germany/fenugreek seeds	O104:H4	2,987 (unknown, 53)
2011	Romaine lettuce	O157:H7	58 (33, 0)

Centers for Disease Control and Prevention. (2018). Reports of selected *E. coli* outbreak investigations. Retrieved from https://www.cdc.gov/ecoli/outbreaks.html

had become a commonly implicated culprit in non-beef outbreaks, including those involving produce (an FDA-regulated product).[18]

The outbreaks in the 1990s and 2000s were publicized, scrutinized, and rapidly shared across the newly arriving, omnipresent tool of social media, and politicians were compelled to act. Key federal governmental and congressional political actors involved in the conceptualizing and eventual authoring of bills to give the FDA new powers for regulating these foodborne pathogens included, but were not limited to, David Acheson (FDA), Sen. Dick Durbin (D-IL), Rep. Rosa DeLauro (D-CT), Rep. John Dingell (D-MI), Rep. Henry Waxman (D-CA), Sen. Jon Tester (D-MT), and Sen. Tom Harkin (D-IA). Bills and amendments appeared in 2008 and 2009, though some politicians were reluctant to lend support to them. The insertion of a "Tester Amendment," which advocated exemptions or delays in implementation for small-scale farmers and producers, made the eventual FSMA bill more palatable to law-makers.[19] The Tester amendment was named for Sen. Jon Tester of Montana, who, along with Sen. Kay Hagan of North Carolina, advocated on behalf of small-scale, organic, and niche food producers.

Having been inaugurated into office 2 years earlier, President Barack Obama signed the FDA Food Safety Modernization Act into law on January 4, 2011. At 89 pages in length, FSMA laid a new plank in the primary-policy foundation for the United States. Since 2011, a number of secondary-policy regulations (or rules) have also been enacted: the Current Good Manufacturing Practice, Hazard Analysis, and Risk-Based Preventive Controls for Human Food rule; the Standards for the Growing, Harvesting, Packing, and Holding of Produce for Human Consumption rule; and the Mitigation Strategies to Protect Food Against Intentional Adulteration rule, among others.[20]

Summary Points

1. FSMA represented the first major overhaul of U.S. food safety law in half a century.
2. CDC surveillance programs (including FoodNet and PulseNet) provided evidence and justification for FSMA and its subsequent regulations.
3. FSMA was birthed from an awareness that pathogens such as *Salmonella* and STEC are not confined to meat products.
4. Highly publicized outbreaks, subsequent liability lawsuits, and social media forces all played a part in Congress passing and President Barack Obama signing FSMA.

▶ Application of CEPH MPH Competencies

This case study addresses CEPH competency 12.

Competency 12: Discuss Multiple Dimensions of the Policy-Making Process, Including the Roles of Ethics and Evidence

Public health policy-making is multidimensional, and the case of FSMA illustrates its complex nature. Different levels and branches of government are responsible for primary policies (i.e., laws) and secondary policies (i.e., regulations). While Congress, with the signature of the president, can bring into force primary laws, myriad Cabinet-level agencies routinely adopt secondary regulations. For example, the USDA's FSIS and the Department of Health and Human Services' FDA routinely adopt regulations, and do so under the authority of congressionally adopted primary laws (e.g., the Federal Meat Inspection Act and the Food Drug and Cosmetic Act). Policy-making's multiple dimensions also appear in the different kinds of actors involved in these processes: bureaucratic policy-makers nested in cabinet agencies, elected politicians in the Congress, and scientists in activist organizations, just to name a few. In FSMA's case, an array of actors made contributions in proposing and passing this important primary law.

In his eight-step policy analysis framework, Eugene Bardach argues that evidence is key to policy-making.[21] Indeed, evidence has served as the cornerstone for FSMA's justification: surveillance demonstrated that outbreaks were increasing, scientific techniques permitted rapid identification of causative agents, and lawmakers received communications from constituents and think tanks demanding policy change. While anecdotal evidence has always been available, it was the CDC's robust surveillance data that ultimately provided convincing evidence to justify the creation of FSMA.[22]

Author Upton Sinclair started the tradition of holding food companies to ethical standards. Ethical standards in food production are important because persons from all walks of life interact with the food system every day, often multiple times, and their expectations are high.[2,23] Consumers expect the foods they purchase to be properly labeled, safe, and exactly what the label purports them to be.[2] As seen in this case study, ethics is closely tied with issues of food safety, particularly those related to microbial contamination: Laws, market incentives, social norms, public health, and microbiological methods and detection all interact to determine how "acceptable safety" is defined. Control and regulation of bacterial contamination of food involve government, industry, and tort liability.[24] Closely related to ethics is liability—that is, the responsibility to pay for damages.[25] Following the events in our case study, liability has been established through *traceability systems* and the ability to *take cases to court*.[24,25] From a traceability perspective, this means the ability to follow a product back to the farm or facility of origin and understand its path through the supply chain to the consumer.[25] Traceability permits companies to shift responsibility along the supply chain if necessary while giving consumers the ability to seek compensation when damages are warranted.[25]

Where should public health policy-makers seek to apply ethical and liability responsibilities: on the food industry, on the government, or on private citizens? The consumption of raw milk is a hotly debated, highly contentious issue in the United States that presents this question. Numerous states permit the sale of raw milk by various means (although it is illegal to sell this product across state lines), such as on-farm sales. Yet, public health evidence has confirmed time and again that unpasteurized milk is a health risk, and the number of outbreaks associated with raw milk consumption trumps those of pasteurized origin.[26] What is the ethical responsibility of a farm selling raw milk? Who is liable if a child loses kidney function following a STEC infection from raw milk purchased by a parent? What about freedom of choice? These questions are the kinds of topics addressed by food ethics.[26,27]

In addition to raw milk, the consumption of raw, ready-to-eat seafood presents liability and ethical issues; popular products, such as sushi and raw oysters, are potential hosts for a variety of pathogenic microorganisms.[28] Additionally, raw sprouts, deemed a high-risk food by FDA, continue to appear on deli menus despite repeated outbreaks associated with their consumption.[29,30] These ethical considerations are important for understanding and application of MPH Foundational Competency 15, "Evaluate policies for their impact on public health and health equity," to ensure that evidence of health risks is carefully considered when crafting new policy.

Discussion Questions

1. What role does public health surveillance (e.g., by the CDC) play in the food safety policy-making process?
2. Political scientists argue that it is easier for a Cabinet-level agency to adopt a secondary policy (e.g., a regulation or rule) than for Congress to pass a primary policy (e.g., a legislative act). Why do you think this is the case?
3. What is the role of the private sector in ethically utilizing retail data to inform policy-making, given that production practices, consumer purchasing patterns (e.g., shoppers' cards), and supply chain information are all valuable sources of information?
4. How should public health officials approach high-risk food products (e.g., raw oysters, raw milk)? Where should the line be drawn between freedom of choice and ensuring public health?

References

1. Johnson, R. (2014). *The federal food safety system: A primer*. Washington, DC: Congressional Research Service.
2. Sanchez, M. C. (2015). Introduction to statutory framework and case law. In M. C. Sanchez (Ed.), *Food law and regulation for non-lawyers: A U.S. perspective* (pp. 2–3). Cham, Switzerland: Springer International Publishing.
3. Centers for Disease Control and Prevention. (2015). Foodborne outbreaks: Key players in foodborne outbreak response. Retrieved from https://www.cdc.gov/foodsafety/outbreaks/investigating-outbreaks/key-players.html
4. World Heath Organization. (2007). Foodborne disease outbreaks: Guidelines for investigation and control, surveillance to detect foodborne disease. Retrieved from http://www.who.int/foodsafety/publications/foodborne_disease/Section_3.pdf
5. Centers for Disease Control and Prevention. (2016). Foodborne Diseases Active Surveillance Network (FoodNet): About FoodNet.. Retrieved from https://www.cdc.gov/foodnet/about.html
6. Centers for Disease Control and Prevention. (2016). PulseNet: Frequently asked questions. Retrieved from https://www.cdc.gov/pulsenet/about/faq.html
7. Centers for Disease Control and Prevention. (2016). Burden of foodborne illness: Findings. Retrieved from https://www.cdc.gov/foodborneburden/index.html
8. Scallan, E., Hoekstra, R. M., Angulo, F. J., Tauxe, R. V., Widdowson, M.-A., Roy, S. L., . . . Griffin, P. M. (2011). Foodborne illness acquired in the United States: Major pathogens. *Emerging Infectious Diseases, 17*(1), 7–15. doi:10.3201/eid1701.P11101
9. Hennessy, T. W., Hedberg, C. W., Slutsker, L., White, K. E., Besser-Wiek, J. M., Moen, M. E., . . . Osterholm, M. T. (1996). A national outbreak of *Salmonella enteritidis* infections from ice cream. *New England Journal of Medicine, 334*(20), 1281–1286. doi:10.1056/nejm199605163342001
10. Porterfield, E., & McClatchy, A. B. (1995, June 17). Jack In The Box ignored food safety regulations, court documents say. *Spokesman-Review*. Retrieved from http://www.spokesman.com/stories/1995/jun/17/jack-in-the-box-ignored-food-safety-regulations/
11. U.S. Department of Agriculture, Food Safety and Inspection Service. (1996). Pathogen reduction: Hazard Analysis and Critical Control Point (HACCP) systems. *Federal Register, 61*(144), 38806–38989.

12. Barton Behravesh, C., Mody, R. K., Jungk, J., Gaul, L., Redd, J. T., Chen, S., . . . Williams, I. T. (2011). 2008 outbreak of *Salmonella* Saintpaul infections associated with raw produce. *New England Journal of Medicine, 364*(10), 918–927. doi:10.1056/NEJMoa1005741

13. Centers for Disease Control and Prevention. (2006). Update on multi-state outbreak of *E. coli* O157:H7 infections from fresh spinach, October 6, 2006. Retrieved from http://www.cdc.gov/ecoli/2006/september/updates/100606.htm

14. Sanchez, M. C. (2015). Private actions and personal liability. In M. C. Sanchez (Ed.), *Food law and regulation for non-lawyers: A U.S. perspective* (pp. 197–231). Cham, Switzerland: Springer International Publishing.

15. Gyles, C. L. (2007). Shiga toxin-producing *Escherichia coli*: An overview. *Journal of Animal Science, 85*(13 suppl), E45–E62. doi:10.2527/jas.2006-508

16. Moore, J. E. (2004). Gastrointestinal outbreaks associated with fermented meats. *Meat Science, 67*(4), 565–568. https://doi.org/10.1016/j.meatsci.2003.12.009

17. Murray, P. R., Rosenthal, K. S., & Pfaller, M. A. (2013). *Enterobacteriaceae medical microbiology* (7th ed.). Philadelphia, PA: Saunders-Elsevier.

18. Centers for Disease Control and Prevention. (2018). Reports of selected *E. coli* outbreak investigations. Retrieved from https://www.cdc.gov/ecoli/outbreaks.html

19. Hassanein, N. (2011). Matters of scale and the politics of the Food Safety Modernization Act. *Agriculture and Human Values, 28*(4), 577–581. doi:10.1007/s10460-011-9338-6

20. Food and Drug Administration. (2018). FDA Food Safety Modernization Act (FSMA) rules and regulated programs. Retrieved from https://www.fda.gov/Food/GuidanceRegulation/FSMA/

21. Bardach, E. (2000). *A practical guide for policy analysis: The eightfold path to more effective problem solving*. New York, NY: Chatham House Publishers of Seven Bridges Press.

22. Fontanazza, M. (2017). Food safety over past 25 years: "Everything has changed." *Food Safety Tech.* Retrieved from https://foodsafetytech.com/news_article/food-safety-past-25-years-everything-changed/

23. Kaiser, M., & Algers, A. (2016). Food ethics: A wide field in need of dialogue. *Food Ethics, 1*(1), 1–7. doi:10.1007/s41055-016-0007-8

24. Lytton, T. D. (2017). The taming of the stew: Regulatory intermediaries in food safety governance. *Annals of the American Academy of Political and Social Science, 670*(1), 78–92. doi:10.1177/0002716217690330

25. Pouliot, S., & Sumner, D. A. (2008). Traceability, liability, and incentives for food safety and quality. *American Journal of Agricultural Economics, 90*(1), 15–27. doi:10.1111/j.1467-8276.2007.01061.x

26. Oliver, S. P., Boor, K. J., Murphy, S. C., & Murinda, S. E. (2009). Food safety hazards associated with consumption of raw milk. *Foodborne Pathogens and Disease, 6*(7), 793–806. doi:10.1089/fpd.2009.0302

27. Yilmaz, T., Moyer, B., MacDonell, R. E., Cordero-Coma, M., & Gallagher, M. J. (2009). Outbreaks associated with unpasteurized milk and soft cheese: An overview of consumer safety. *Food Protection Trends, 29*(4), 211–222.

28. Kim, H. W., Hong, Y. J., Jo, J. I., Ha, S. D., Kim, S. H., Lee, H. J., & Rhee, M. S. (2017). Raw ready-to-eat seafood safety: Microbiological quality of the various seafood species available in fishery, hyper and online markets. *Letters in Applied Microbiology, 64*(1), 27–34. doi:10.1111/lam.12688

29. Callejon, R. M., Rodriguez-Naranjo, M. I., Ubeda, C., Hornedo-Ortega, R., Garcia-Parrilla, M. C., & Troncoso, A. M. (2015). Reported foodborne outbreaks due to fresh produce in the United States and European Union: Trends and causes. *Foodborne Pathogens and Disease, 12*(1), 32–38. doi:10.1089/fpd.2014.1821

30. Food and Drug Administration. (2018). FSMA final rule on produce safety. Retrieved from https://www.fda.gov/food/guidanceregulation/fsma/ucm334114.htm

CHAPTER 13

Within "REACH": Community–Campus Partnership to Support Research, Education, and Community Health

Cara L. Pennel, DrPH, MPH
John D. Prochaska, DrPH, MPH
Neilson Treble, LPC, ACPS
Rob Ruffner, MPA
Sharon Croisant, PhD, MS

▶ Background

Community Coalitions Defined

Community coalitions and partnerships have become integral to public health approaches to improving health. Coalitions are groups of individual or organizational stakeholders, oftentimes representing different sectors, who join together for a common cause or goal, frequently to address an identified health or social issue.[1-3] The sectors involved in coalitions may depend on the area of focus, but often include public health, other local government, nonprofit organizations, health care, businesses, education (public, private, and higher), law enforcement, grassroots organizations, faith-based groups, and concerned citizens.[4-6]

Why Are Community Coalitions Important?

Community-based health promotion and disease prevention efforts have used coalitions and partnerships to address a broad range of issues, including tobacco control,[5,7,8] alcohol and substance abuse,[7,9-12] teen pregnancy prevention,[7,13,14] asthma,[15,16] chronic disease,[5] violence and crime prevention,[10,11] environmental hazards,[17,18] domestic violence,[18] racism,[18] deteriorating housing and neighborhoods,[18] access to health care,[19] and economic development.[18] Coalitions' diversity in composition brings a broad range of voices and perspectives to bear on a common issue, allowing the collective framing of an issue that can be understood and, ultimately, addressed using points of view, expertise, and resources that span sectoral boundaries.

While coalitions *can* provide health education and influence individual behaviors, an advantage of the diverse representation and talents of community coalitions is the potential for health impact at a greater, population-based level.[20] In fact, coalitions may build on and expand existing education and individual behavior change efforts.[21] Such expansions might involve advocating for change. Advocacy efforts can be directed toward local and state policy-makers to influence and develop policy, or toward local businesses and organizations to change practices. Coalitions can advocate for changes to the environment, including the built environment, such as making neighborhoods safer and more conducive for physical activity, and the social environment, such as creating opportunities for youth or cultural development.[22,23]

Generally, participants in community coalitions have a good sense of what is happening "on the ground" in their community as well as which strategies would be most appropriate and effective for their community. Coalitions may organize around a specific, local issue of concern (e.g., industrialized hog farming in rural North Carolina)[17] or larger national issues that a community feels compelled to address locally (e.g., access to quality health care for uninsured populations), or they may take on multiple health or social issues at multiple ecological levels.

Working jointly together for change, coalitions may be able to tackle community issues that are too large and complex for any one agency or organization to confront alone. Coalitions can facilitate pooling of limited community resources, such as funding and personnel[22,24]; emphasize a strengths-based approach using existing assets[5]; and minimize the duplication of efforts.[22] Finally, community coalitions can help garner public support for identified issues, enhance local ownership and community buy-in, promote sustainability, and support dissemination and implementation.[12]

▶ Case Study

This case study discusses strategies to identify stakeholders and build coalitions and partnerships to influence health outcomes, using the Galveston County Research, Education, And Community Health (REACH) community coalition as an example.

In 2014, the REACH coalition was formed by a small group consisting of six community organization leaders and six University of Texas Medical Branch (UTMB) researchers and educators in Galveston County, Texas. These 12 stakeholders came together initially to discuss forming a "coalition of coalitions" that could serve as a common advisory board for both community organizations and academic institutions. The rationale was that this single group could simplify communication and reduce the burden for faculty and community service groups, which were often over-committed and under-resourced. We soon found that our meetings provided valuable opportunities to share information and explore the possibilities of community–campus partnerships to improve understanding of community issues and better address them collaboratively.

Broadly, the purpose of REACH is to build community and academic partnerships to address the diverse public health needs and opportunities in Galveston County. REACH does this by sharing information and resources among nonprofit, governmental, and academic entities; developing and vetting programs, materials, and best practices for replication and dissemination; providing a forum for brokering relationships among member partners to align efforts toward common goals; addressing the needs of Galveston County by minimizing gaps and duplicated services/efforts; and leveraging time, funding, human resources, and efforts. Currently, the REACH coalition is composed of approximately 40 Galveston County nonprofit organization/governmental agency representatives and 20 university department, center, and institute representatives at three higher education institutions. The general REACH membership meets quarterly.

The REACH Executive Committee is composed of 11 partner representatives, 6 community and 5 academic, who meet monthly to discuss and direct more logistical and operational issues that arise in keeping the coalition moving forward. Leadership positions within the Executive Committee are identified as the Chair, Past Chair, Vice Chair, and Secretary. The Chair position alternates annually between community and academic partners. For example, the current past Chair (inaugural REACH chair), is a community representative, the current Chair is an academic representative, and the Vice Chair is a community representative. Each serves a 1-year term before moving to the next higher position (e.g., the Vice Chair becomes the Chair, and the Chair becomes the Past Chair). The Secretary serves a 2-year term. In addition to the Executive Committee, REACH is also organized into a series of work groups formed around particular projects of interest to portions of the membership. Current work groups include a Community Health Needs Assessment Work Group, a Bylaws and Membership Work Group, an Advocacy Work Group, a Strategic Planning Work Group, and a Community-Based Participatory Research Work Group. These work groups report their progress to the broader membership during the regular general meeting and Executive Committee.

Achievements and Successes

In addition to the completion of the county-wide community health needs assessment (discussed later in this case study), another key achievement of REACH is a youth risk behavior survey that has been completed at the local high school biannually. Modeled on the Centers for Disease Control and Prevention's (CDC) Youth Risk Behavior Surveillance Survey (YRBSS), this survey provides evidence and strategic direction for community and academic partners working with youth. For example, the 2014 youth survey indicated nearly half of all ninth- through twelfth-grade students (44.7%) were sexually active, and 20% reported having sexual intercourse before the age of 13. Of sexually active students, one in six reported they had been pregnant or gotten someone pregnant. In response, a master of public health (MPH) student/general preventive medicine resident worked with the Galveston County Health District and other community partners to develop and implement an adolescent pregnancy prevention program plan as her applied practice experience. In conjunction with her practice experience, her capstone project (integrative learning experience) involved creating and conducting an evaluation plan for the program.

Another REACH accomplishment since 2014 is brokering approximately 25 applied practice experiences and community-based practice projects for MPH students with local organizations and agencies. Each general membership meeting includes an "offer and ask" session. During this time, the Public Health Program at UTMB has the opportunity to offer the assistance of one or more MPH students to work on community-based practice projects, and community organizations have the opportunity to ask for student assistance on projects within their organization. These often include program planning, program evaluation, or data analysis and reporting. Past project examples have included implementing a healthy food inventory system and policies with the Galveston County Food Bank, conducting descriptive analysis of disease outbreaks with the Galveston County Health District, developing and implementing nutrition education curriculum for children with Galveston Urban Ministries, designing a survey of needed services and an accompanying database with a local social service nonprofit organization, preparing numerous nonprofit organizations for disasters with Galveston County Mutual Assistance Partnership (GC-MAP), and working with a Galveston Police sergeant and GC-MAP to conduct workplace violence assessments and make recommendations to improve organizational staff and client safety.

REACH has completed bylaws and submitted the coalition's application to become a 501(c)3 organization. Being formally designated as a nonprofit organization gives the coalition the ability to seek and apply for funding for which individual member organizations may not individually be eligible. REACH is also involved in a strategic planning process with community and academic partner engagement, using the community health needs assessment, youth survey, and membership organization foci, to determine what priority areas the coalition will pursue over the next 3 years.

Summary Points

1. The Galveston County REACH coalition was formed to influence health outcomes and create change within the respective communities that the coalition's member organizations serve.

2. The coalition serves as an excellent avenue for resource sharing and has created additional opportunities for collaboration among members that might not have otherwise been discovered.

3. Through future endeavors, such as obtaining status as a 501(c)3 organization and the Community-Based Participatory Research work group, the REACH coalition intends to further push for interaction and cooperation between academic and community partners, including expansion of past efforts such as the youth survey and community health needs assessment.

▶ Application of CEPH MPH Competencies

This case study addresses CEPH competencies 13, 2, and 4.

Competency 13: Propose Strategies to Identify Stakeholders and Build Coalitions and Partnerships for Influencing Public Health Outcomes

Beyond the initial group of community and university leaders, REACH membership grew largely based on stakeholder interest in two priorities identified by the coalition: the need to conduct a comprehensive community health needs assessment (CHNA) and the collective desire to develop a broad-based series of educational trainings related to community-based research. REACH membership became open, inclusive, and dynamic, garnering broad-based, high-impact community participation, including public and mental health agencies, clinicians, policy-makers from local governmental and quasi-governmental bodies, family services centers, cultural and faith-based organizations, other nonprofit organizations, and local schools and colleges.

While initiating the coalition was greatly facilitated by working on these two common projects, REACH leadership recognized early in the process that, despite the enthusiasm for building the coalition, we would need to continually address several important issues: fostering relationships of trust and equity, establishing true partnerships, and reducing—if not eliminating—the power differential between academia and community organizations. These realizations fostered the establishment of bylaws and the application for independent, nonprofit status, which further reinforced the process of building trusting relationships.

Competency 2: Select Quantitative and Qualitative Data Collection Methods Appropriate for a Given Public Health Context

An early priority of REACH was to develop and maintain a robust database of key population health indicators, population health-related needs, and available resources for the broader Galveston County population. Earlier work involved collecting qualitative data for subgroups, such as interviewing and conducting focus groups with low-income residents or specific neighborhoods severely affected by natural disasters (e.g., Hurricane Ike). While the qualitative data helped provide guidance for the next steps (e.g., survey methodology, question/instrument development, population oversampling), no single effort had collected quantitative data on the population as a whole. The CHNA Work Group was formed and reached consensus on the types of quantitative community data needed, including general health status; morbidity; access to health services, food, transportation, and employment; health behaviors; needed and utilized community-based resources; demographics; and neighborhood perceptions. The Work Group mailed paper surveys to a random sample of county households, using a commercially available address database (with the option to complete the survey online). We selected this approach based on input from both academic and community stakeholders. Limited resources precluded translation of the survey into multiple languages, and the returned surveys reflected this limitation.

Competency 4: Interpret Results of Data Analysis for Public Health Research, Policy, or Practice

The CHNA survey data were analyzed and the results were vetted with the CHNA Work Group to ensure the findings were congruent with what both academic and community partners expected. Informational presentations and one-page briefs were developed around specific audience interests for dissemination of the findings to key partners. For example, CHNA faculty and staff presented data on alcohol, drugs, and tobacco to the Bay Area Council on Drugs and Alcohol for use in grants. Broader health findings were distributed to local philanthropic foundations to aid in strategic planning and funding priority decisions as well as more specific products around adverse childhood experiences, food insecurity, and disaster preparedness. In each case, interpretation and translation of results was a participatory process, wherein both academic and community members provided input. This further enhanced the relevancy and facilitated uptake of information to those who requested it.

The CHNA process provided a population-wide assessment of a broad range of population health indicators around disease and condition incidence and prevalence, resources available and utilized, needs, and broader indicators, such as neighborhood- and community-level quality indicators. The results from this process have been used within REACH to set priorities in forming new work groups, bring attention to previously unrealized issues, and provide a baseline against which to measure and evaluate impact of various efforts aimed at improving population health. The CHNA process helped to broaden the impact, beyond community and academic settings, to local and regional policy-making arenas.

Discussion Questions

1. What is the composition of the REACH coalition? Which sectors do you think should be invited to the table if the focus were teen pregnancy prevention? Access to mental health services? Preventing gun violence? Which sectors would you want involved no matter the issue?
2. What are the advantages and disadvantages of very broad community representation on the coalition? What are the advantages and disadvantages of narrower community representation?
3. Every coalition must find its own balance between the process of coalition building and action toward outcomes. What might be some challenges balancing process and action? How would you handle these challenges?
4. Research suggests community partnerships are essential for creating effective and sustainable public health programs. Why might these partnerships be necessary to create effective programs? Why are they necessary to create sustainable programs?

References

1. Alexander, J. A., Comfort, M. E., Weiner, B. J., & Bogue, R. (2001). Leadership in collaborative community health partnerships. *Nonprofit Management and Leadership, 12*(2), 159–175. doi:10.1002/nml.12203

2. Berkowitz, W. R., & Wolff, T. (2000). *The spirit of the coalition.* Washington, DC: American Public Health Association.

3. Feighery, E., & Rogers, T. (1995). *Building and maintaining effective coalitions.* Palo Alto, CA: Health Promotion Resource Center.

4. Brown, L. D., Wells, R., Jones, E. C., & Chilenski, S. M. (2017). Effects of sectoral diversity on community coalition processes and outcomes. *Prevention Science, 18*(5), 600–609. doi:10.1007/s11121-017-0796-y

5. Butterfoss, F. D., Goodman, R. M., & Wandersman, A. (1996). Community coalitions for prevention and health promotion: Factors predicting satisfaction, participation, and planning. *Health Education Quarterly, 23*(1), 65–79. doi:10.1177/109019819602300105

6. Zakocs, R. C., & Edwards, E. M. (2006). What explains community coalition effectiveness? *American Journal of Preventive Medicine, 30*(4), 351–361. doi:10.1016/j.amepre.2005.12.004

7. Foster-Fishman, P. G., Berkowitz, S. L., Lounsbury, D. W., Jacobson, S., & Allen, N. A. (2001). Building collaborative capacity in community coalitions: A review and integrative framework. *American Journal of Community Psychology, 29*(2), 241–261. doi:10.1023/a:1010378613583

8. Kegler, M. C., Steckler, A., Mcleroy, K., & Malek, S. H. (1998). Factors that contribute to effective community health promotion coalitions: A study of 10 Project ASSIST coalitions in North Carolina. *Health Education & Behavior, 25*(3), 338–353. doi:10.1177/109019819802500308

9. Fawcett, S. B., Lewis, R. K., Paine-Andrews, A., Francisco, V. T., Richter, K. P., Williams, E. L., & Copple, B. (1997). Evaluating community coalitions for prevention of substance abuse: The case of Project Freedom. *Health Education & Behavior, 24*(6), 812–828. doi:10.1177/109019819702400614

10. Feinberg, M. E., Jones, D., Greenberg, M. T., Osgood, D. W., & Bontempo, D. (2010). Effects of the Communities That Care model in Pennsylvania on change in adolescent risk and problem behaviors. *Prevention Science, 11,* 163–171.

11. Hawkins, J. D., Oesterle, S., Brown, E. C., Arthur, M. W., Abbott, R. D., Fagan, A. A., & Catalano, R. F. (2009). Results of a type 2 translational research trial to prevent adolescent drug use and delinquency: A test of Communities That Care. *Archives of Pediatric and Adolescent Medicine, 163,* 789–798.

12. Flewelling, R. L., & Hanley, S. M. (2016). Assessing community coalition capacity and its association with underage drinking prevention effectiveness in the context of the SPF SIG. *Prevention Science, 17*(7), 830–840. doi:10.1007/s11121-016-0675-y

13. Kegler, M. C., Williams, C. W., Cassell, C. M., Santelli, J., Kegler, S. R., Montgomery, S. B., . . . Hunt, S. C. (2005). Mobilizing communities for teen pregnancy prevention: Associations between coalition characteristics and perceived accomplishments. *Journal of Adolescent Health, 37*(3). doi:10.1016/j.jadohealth.2005.05.011

14. Kramer, J. S., Philliber, S., Brindis, C. D., Kamin, S. L., Chadwick, A. E., Revels, M. L., . . . Valderrama, L. T. (2005). Coalition models: Lessons learned from the CDC's Community Coalition Partnership Programs for the Prevention of Teen Pregnancy. *Journal of Adolescent Health, 37*(3). doi:10.1016/j.jadohealth.2005.05.010

15. Butterfoss, F. D., Kelly, C., & Taylor-Fishwick, J. (2005). Health planning that magnifies the community's voice: Allies Against Asthma. *Health Education & Behavior, 32*(1), 113–128. doi:10.1177/1090198104269568

16. Clark, N., Doctor, L., Friedman, A., Lachance, L., Houle, C., Geng, X., & Grisso, J. (2006). Community coalitions to control chronic disease: Allies Against Asthma as a model and case study. *Health Promotion Practice, 7*(2), 13S–22S.

17. Policy Link. (n.d.). Promoting healthy public policy through community-based participatory research: Ten case studies. Retrieved from http://www.policylink.org/resources-tools/promoting-healthy-public-policy-through-community-based-participatory-research-ten-case-studies

18. Wolff, T. (2001). Community coalition building: Contemporary practice and research: Introduction. *American Journal of Community Psychology, 29*(2), 165–172. doi:10.1023/a:1010314326787

19. Bibeau, D. L., Howell, K. A., Rife, J. C., & Taylor, M. L. (1996). The role of a community coalition in the development of health services for the poor and uninsured. *International Journal of Health Services, 26*(1), 93–110. doi:10.2190/T3RN-0578-6U4M-CNNN

20. Frieden, T. R. (2010). A framework for public health action: The health impact pyramid. *American Journal of Public Health, 100*(4), 590–595. doi:10.2105/ajph.2009.185652

21. Wolff, T. (2001). The future of community coalition building. *American Journal of Community Psychology, 29*(2), 263–268. doi:10.1023/a:1010330730421

22. Center for Community Health and Development, Community Tool Box. (2018). Chapter 5, Section 5: Coalition building I: Starting a coalition. Lawrence, KS: University of Kansas. Retrieved from https://ctb.ku.edu/en/table-of-contents/assessment/promotion-strategies/start-a-coalition/main

23. Roussos, S. T., & Fawcett, S. B. (2000). A review of collaborative partnerships as a strategy for improving community health. *Annual Review of Public Health, 20*, 369–402.

24. Kegler, M. C., & Swan, D. W. (2011). Advancing coalition theory: The effect of coalition factors on community capacity mediated by member engagement. *Health Education Research, 27*(4), 572–584. doi:10.1093/her/cyr083

CHAPTER 14

Photovoice as a Tool for Change: Engaging the Community in Public Health Advocacy

Suzanne Carlberg-Racich, PhD, MSPH

▶ Background

The opioid epidemic has become an issue of national significance in the United States due to increases in overdose mortality,[1] a growing awareness of the role of prescription opioids in the crisis,[2] and changing demographics for individuals using opioids.[3] While not the main focus of the national media, people who inject drugs (PWID), particularly heroin, have been dying from overdose for decades. Efforts to reduce overdose and other injection-related harms have stemmed mostly from grassroots harm-reduction programs. These programs have been successful in reducing risks from the sharing of injection equipment,[4,5] reducing HIV transmission,[6,7] reducing hepatitis transmission,[8] connecting clients to treatment,[9,10] and reducing overdose rates through the distribution of naloxone (Narcan®), an opioid overdose-reversal agent.[11]

While overdose prevention and treatment has recently been prioritized as a target for federal funding, efforts to reduce other injection risks remain subject to politically charged decision making. For example, a federal ban on funding for syringes persists, despite decades of evidence and seven U.S. government-funded investigations of syringe exchange programs that all demonstrated the provision of injection equipment prevents the spread of infection without increasing drug use.[12] Similarly, the more recent outbreak of HIV transmission in Scott County, Indiana, has illustrated how quickly viral transmission can occur in the absence of these critical services, yet local politicians continue to challenge efforts to distribute life-saving injection supplies.

While syringe programs serve a critical role in preventing HIV, hepatitis, and other infections, they cannot fully address the harms associated with public injection. The legal harms associated with possessing and using heroin leave PWID unable to engage in a safer, more sterile injection process. This is exacerbated for those who are homeless or precariously housed, who lack a clean and private space to inject, and who face the risk of impending arrest while injecting outside or in restaurant bathrooms. Other countries have addressed these harms by providing safe consumption spaces (SCS)—that is, places where PWID can obtain sterile equipment, inject in a safe, clean environment, and be monitored for overdose without worry of arrest. Evidence from a myriad of programs has demonstrated benefits from such practices, including reductions in overdose and emergency services utilization for overdose in communities surrounding SCS,[13] facilitation of treatment and reduction in drug use,[14] a decrease in public injection, and no change in crime.[15] Thus, the opposition to SCS tends to wane after their successful implementation.[16]

While SCS has received local approval in a few cities recently, sanctioned programs have yet to be implemented in the United States and remain an issue of political debate. Where advocacy efforts exist, they are mainly led by harm-reduction organizations, community organizers, and a few drug-user union groups. Perhaps the most significant barrier to advocacy efforts is the lack of consistent and widespread PWID voice. This is due to the overwhelming stigma and potential legal and social repercussions from publicly declaring oneself to be a PWID. PWID experience ongoing pervasive sigma,[17] and this stigma is associated with poor health outcomes.[18] While efforts to unionize PWID are of critical importance, alternative opportunities are also needed to give PWID a voice. The project described in this case study provided a safer option to inform advocacy efforts, using a method called Photovoice.

Photovoice was originally developed to empower people to identify community assets and deficits through use of photography, and to use the photos to improve awareness and policy.[19] With this method, community members take photos to illustrate issues and provide narratives to aid in telling the story. The option for participants to select their own images allows them to remain anonymous if they so choose and provides a safe alternative to common advocacy efforts such as testifying before local officials. Thus, it is an ideal fit to fill the advocacy gap for PWID.

▶ Case Study

This project was a collaboration between an academic institution and a harm-reduction program operating in an urban area. The primary aims were to (1) engage and train PWID in telling stories about the value of harm-reduction services with photography and narratives, and (2) use the photos and narratives to influence local policy. Rather than advocating based on public health data or evidence, the project engendered an exploration of the meaning, depth, and value of the services to PWID.

The project team, composed of academic partners and harm-reduction volunteers, met with clients of the harm-reduction program to obtain guidance on how to structure the project. Clients articulated the need for questions to guide the process and created a draft with assistance from the project team. The questions included asking participants why they seek harm-reduction services, the benefits they receive from those services, and what else they need to stay safe. Project participants were recruited from outreach vans in areas with high incidence of opioid overdose, with purposeful variation in gender identification, racial/ethnic background, and age. Interested participants were engaged in training on Photovoice, and asked to return with photos within 2 weeks. Upon their return, participants were asked why they took each photo, what they hoped people would learn from it, and how the photos might be used to change policy.

A total of 24 participants completed the study and returned with photos, with a combined total of 80 photos. The photos were grouped by question and reviewed by the team to draft a codebook. Following that, the photos and narrative were coded independently by three members of the team. The team then met to review concordant and discordant coding and to discuss emergent themes. Photos representing each theme were printed together and presented to participants for member checking, to ensure the authenticity of themes generated by the team.

Access to Life and Health

Several themes emerged from the photos and narrative. The most prevalent theme—the fundamental need to stay healthy and the limited service options to support that need—is the focus of this case study. Participants discussed the difficulties of obtaining safer injection equipment and other necessities, citing discrimination and cost as barriers to pharmacy purchase, and applauding harm-reduction programs as a way to access these things that they could not access or afford elsewhere. **FIGURES 14-1** and **14-2** illustrate this theme.

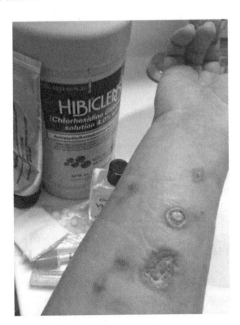

FIGURE 14-1 I come to the van because these wounds would be a lot worse without the services provided by the van. The risks from injecting are reduced a great deal by getting education and the tools to inject in a safer way.

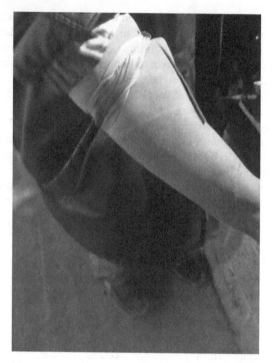

FIGURE 14-2 I need these services to get my supplies: needles, cookers, water, and tie string. These things keep me safe and keep the arm safe. This way I don't tear my skin and I no longer have war wounds.
Courtesy of Suzanne Carlberg-Racich.

This need for safety extended beyond the individual to their families, friends, and communities. Participants talked about the importance of staying healthy and alive for partners and children. They also talked about protecting their families and communities from contaminated syringes, and that the harm reduction program was their only option, as home disposal would put others at risk. They photographed methods of safe transport back to the van, including hard-sided soda bottles or sharps containers provided by their local program, and the need to prevent others from acquiring infections (**FIGURE 14-3**).

The theme of access to health and life extended to other program services, including vaccinations and testing that are cost prohibitive elsewhere, and naloxone to prevent overdose death. Access to naloxone was a prevalent theme in itself, with participants describing how they revived friends from overdose death as a result of the program (**FIGURE 14-4**).

They also highlighted the importance of this medication in saving their own lives (**FIGURE 14-5**).

Photos and discussion also demonstrated the severity of the consequences if someone did not have access, as conceptualized by **FIGURE 14-6**.

The photos and quotes in Figures 14-4, 14-5, and 14-6 were used in local advocacy efforts in response to the overdose crisis. The academic partner was invited to testify to the municipal opioid task force in preparation for their recommendations to address overdose mortality. The printed testimony contained four policy "priorities"

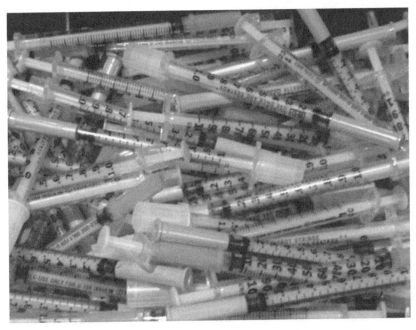

FIGURE 14-3 The [harm-reduction program] is a place to safely discard used supplies to protect the public and the individual from disease.

Courtesy of Suzanne Carlberg-Racich.

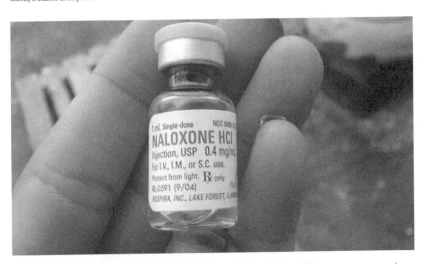

FIGURE 14-4 There is nowhere else that I can get this and I have used it to save someone's life—that's important.

Courtesy of Suzanne Carlberg-Racich.

for the task force to consider, along with these photos and quotes to tell the story of the value of naloxone in the PWID community. Three of the four priorities have been implemented: the allocation of funding for overdose in community-based naloxone distribution programs, explicit requirements for licensed treatment facilities

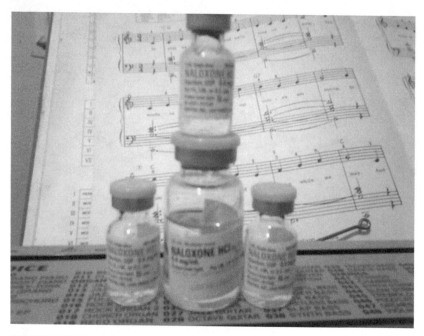

FIGURE 14-5 This has helped me when I've been ODing and I have used it with other people. I want to live so that I can keep playing my music and live a long life.

Courtesy of Suzanne Carlberg-Racich.

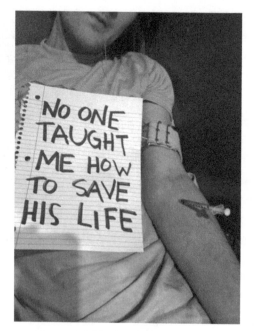

FIGURE 14-6 The program teaches users how to respond to and act in the event of an overdose. This includes handing out naloxone for free.

Courtesy of Suzanne Carlberg-Racich.

to address overdose with naloxone upon discharge, and targeted education efforts to address critical gaps on a citywide basis. While their testimony was not solely responsible for these decisions, participants are proud of their contributions to achieving greater access to this lifesaving medication.

Summary Points

1. Despite national attention to the overdose epidemic, the health needs of PWID are underrepresented, especially injection-related harms.
2. While harm-reduction services and safe consumption spaces demonstrate evidence of public health efficacy, they are hindered by unstable funding and political dissension.
3. PWID are often silenced from traditional advocacy efforts due to stigma and fear of legal repercussions, making it difficult to bring a human voice to these issues.
4. Photovoice presents an alternative, safer option for PWID to participate in advocacy.
5. PWID in this project argue that harm-reduction services are a gateway to safety, better health, and life. Their contributions were a critical part of a successful effort to increase access to lifesaving medication at the municipal level.

▶ Application of CEPH MPH Competencies

This case study addresses CEPH competencies 14 and 6.

Competency 14: Advocate for Political, Social, or Economic Policies and Programs that Will Improve Health in Diverse Populations

This project illustrates the potential for Photovoice to empower local under-represented groups to safely advocate for their unmet needs, and to successfully influence political, social, or economic policies that improve health. While evidence of harm-reduction program efficacy has existed for many years, PWID voice in advocacy efforts has been minimal due to fear and stigma. Facilitating options to integrate the voice of PWID with existing evidence will ensure that those persons who need services are part of the creation of policies and programs that are effective and meaningful.

This case study illustrated the use of photos and narratives from PWID to influence local economic policy related to naloxone funding, targeted education, and licensing requirements. The project yielded 80 photos with accompanying narratives that can inform future efforts and instill a human voice into the policy-making process.

An emerging political debate is focusing on the push for safer consumption spaces in the United States. While vocal harm-reduction groups, public health experts, and others have presented evidence of SCS's efficacy, a stronger PWID voice is needed to illustrate the human impact of policy change. Groups that have strong lobbies of personally affected individuals can engender greater critical consciousness about the human experience. Public health practitioners should create opportunities for systematically disconnected or under-represented groups to participate in advocacy efforts through Photovoice.

Competency 6: Discuss the Means by Which Structural Bias, Social Inequities, and Racism Undermine Health and Create Challenges to Achieving Health Equity at Organizational, Community, and Societal Levels

Inspiration for this project was found in the overwhelming inequities faced by PWID, and the lack of compassion demonstrated toward those individuals by society and its institutions. A pervasive, dangerous stigma distorts efforts to assist PWID, resulting in punitive approaches that further exacerbate the divide between people in need and people who might help. This stigma exists in the very institutions designed to treat substance use disorder—the medical system, corrections, social services, and society at large—resulting in isolation of this population. The voices of PWID need to be heard for this situation to change.

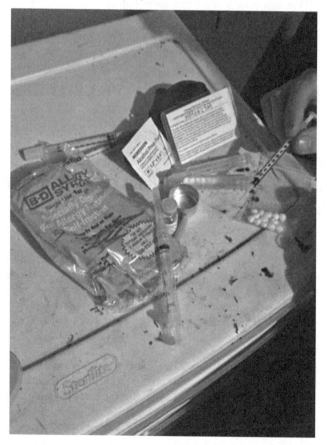

FIGURE 14-7 Unsafe drug using conditions.
Courtesy of Suzanne Carlberg-Racich.

Discussion Questions

1. How might you use the image in **FIGURE 14-7** to advocate for safe consumption spaces in your local area? Which alternatives to printed testimony do you suggest to sway local politicians?

2. If you were to use Photovoice to engage other groups who use drugs (not PWID), which issue would you address? How would you recruit participants? How would you use the results?

3. If you wanted to increase the role of PWID in this project, which other tasks might they engage in to achieve a more participatory approach?

4. What other under-represented and stigmatized groups might benefit from a Photovoice project to advocate for their own health needs? How would you initiate a partnership with the group you suggest?

References

1. Puja, S., Scholl, L., Rudd, R., & Bacon, S. (2018). Overdose deaths involving opioids, cocaine, and psychostimulants—United States, 2015–2016. *Morbidity and Mortality Weekly Report, 67*(12), 349–358.

2. Manchikanti, L., Standiford, H., Fellows, B., Janata, J., Pampati, V., Grider, J., & Boswell, M. (2012). Opioid epidemic in the United States. *Pain Physician, 15,* ES9–ES38.

3. Hanson, H., & Netherland, J. (2016). Is the prescription opioid epidemic a white problem? *American Journal of Public Health, 106*(12), 2127–2129.

4. Heimer, R. (1998). Syringe exchange programs: Lowering the transmission of syringe-borne diseases and beyond. *Public Health Reports, 113,* 67.

5. Hagan, H., DesJarlais, D., Friedman, S., Purchase, D., & Alter, M. (1995). Reduced risk of hepatitis B and hepatitis C among injection drug users in the Tacoma syringe exchange program. *American Journal of Public Health, 85,* 1531.

6. DesJarlais, D., Asareth, K., Hagan, H., McKnight, C., Perlman, D., & Friedman, S. (2009). Persistence and change in disparities in HIV infection among injection drug users in New York City after large-scale syringe exchange programs. *American Journal of Public Health, 99*(S2), S445.

7. DesJarlais, D., Perlis, T., Friedman, S., Deren, S., Chapman, T., Sotheran, J., . . . Marmor, M. (1998). Declining seroprevalence in a very large HIV epidemic: Injecting drug users in New York City, 1991 to 1996. *American Journal of Public Health, 88,* 1801.

8. DesJarlais, D., Perlis, T., Arasteh, K., Torian, L., Hagan, H., Beatrice, S., . . . Friedman, S. (2005). Reductions in hepatitis C virus and HIV infections among injecting drug users in New York City, 1990–2001. *AIDS, 19,* S20.

9. Brooner, R., Kidorf, M., King, V., Beilenson, P., Svikis, D., & Vlahov, D. (1998). Drug abuse treatment success among needle exchange participants. *Public Health Reports, 113*(S1), 129.

10. Hagan, H., McGough, J., Thiede, H., Hopkins, S., Duchin, J., & Alexander, E. (2000). Reduced injection frequency and increased entry and retention in drug treatment associated with needle-exchange participation in Seattle drug injectors. *Journal of Substance Abuse Treatment, 19,* 247.

11. Wheeler, E., Davidson, P., Jones, T., & Irwin, K. (2012). Community-based opioid overdose prevention programs providing naloxone—United States, 2010. *Morbidity and Mortality Weekly Report, 61*(6), 101–105.

12. Satcher, D. (1998). *Evidence-based findings on the efficacy of syringe exchange programs: An analysis of the scientific research completed since April 1998.* Washington, DC: U.S. Department of Health and Human Services.

13. Marshall, B., Milloy, M., Wood, E., Montaner, J., & Kerr, T. (2011). Reduction in overdose mortality after the opening of North America's first medically supervised safer injecting facility: A retrospective population-based study. *Lancet, 377*(9775), 1429–1437.

14. Committee MMSICE. (2003). *Final report of the evaluation of the Sydney Medically Supervised Injection Centre.* Sydney, Australia: MSIC Evaluation Committee.

15. Donnelly, N., & Mahoney, N. (2013). Trends in property and illicit drug crime around the Medically Supervised Injecting Centre in Kings Cross: 2012 update. Retrieved from https://www.bocsar.nsw.gov.au/Documents/BB/bb90.pdf

16. Salmon, A., Thein, H., Kimber, J., Kaldor, J., & Maher, L. (2007). Five years on: What are the community perceptions of drug-related public amenity following the establishment of the Sydney Medically Supervised Injecting Centre? *International Journal on Drug Policy, 18*(1), 46–53.

17. Ware, N., Wyatt, M., & Tugenberg, T. (2005). Social relationships, stigma and adherence to antiretroviral therapy for HIV/AIDS. *AIDS Care, 18*, 904.

18. Ahern, J., Stuber, J., & Galea, S. (2007). Stigma, discrimination and the health of illicit drug users. *Drug and Alcohol Dependence, 88*, 188.

19. Wang, C., & Burris, M. (1007). Photovoice: Concept, methodology, and use for participatory needs assessment. *Health Education and Behavior, 24*(3), 369–387.

CHAPTER 15

Health Equity in the Aftermath of a Natural Disaster

Mark E. Gebhart, MD, FAAEM

▶ Background

Vulnerable populations exist.[1] The literature has identified numerous vulnerable populations, including those at extremes of age, those who suffer from mental health conditions, and those living in poverty. These vulnerable populations often suffer from a lack of health equity, ranging from access to primary and specialty care, preventive medicine, and affordable pharmaceuticals, to inadequate housing and shelter. The lack of adequate housing and shelter can lead to a host of adverse health and social impacts. Homelessness has been identified as a particular risk for those persons affected by mental health disorders. Individuals who are homeless are often adversely impacted by poor and inadequate nutrition, chronic health conditions, substance abuse issues such as tobacco dependence, and drug addiction and dependence.

In the event of a disaster in a community, it is necessary for emergency managers and planners as well as public health practitioners to take into account and to assess needs of the mental health community. The components of the mental health community include housing, inpatient care, and community-based programs. Individuals living in a wide variety of housing and inpatient settings have been the source of significant concern during disasters. This population is often not mobile due to lack of transportation, external support mechanisms, legal considerations, and other mobility-limiting conditions. Without the ability to move and relocate, these individuals must rely upon caregivers, emergency managers, and planners to develop and put in place adequate plans to ensure limited disruptions in their activities of daily living, ensure access to health and medical care, and provide safe and reliably constant shelter and housing during a disaster.[2]

In the aftermath of consequential and catastrophic disasters, including both natural and human-made disasters, planning has taken on new urgency and has been addressed at the federal, state, and local levels. Public health has been included at every level of planning.[3,4] Public health agencies have been charged with the responsibility of ensuring policies are put into place that lead to health equity. Vulnerable populations, also identified as special needs populations, have attracted substantial attention during this planning process. Resources have been identified and, importantly, funding secured to drive the complex and costly assurances established for vulnerable populations.

The state of Mississippi was impacted by Hurricane Katrina in the late summer of 2005. In the immediate aftermath of the hurricane, federal, state, and local leaders turned their attention to identified gaps in plans, procedures, and policies as related to hurricanes, and in broader terms to all-hazards disaster planning.[5] This kind of all-hazards disaster planning is essential for health equity, so that the needs of all individuals and members of every community are addressed. In particular, specific and focused attention is directed toward the special needs populations.

The Mississippi Department of Mental Health (DMH) published the state's disaster preparedness and response plan to address an identified need of the mental health community.[6] This effort was broadly part of nationally driven initiatives to assure health equity for the mental health community. The DMH, which was established in 1974, provides a network of services to persons who experience mental illness, alcohol and/or drug abuse dependency, or mental retardation or developmental disabilities. These services include numerous facilities and community-based programs. During any sort of disaster, the DMH has the identified role of coordinating response activities of all facilities so that safety and health of individuals are assured. The DMH plan is broad and complex and includes specific policies. A key and important policy is sheltering in place. During Hurricane Katrina, adverse health and medical consequences for DMH-served populations emerged as substantive issues, leading to a lack of health equity for these vulnerable populations.

▶ Case Study

Hurricane Katrina was a destructive and deadly Category 5 hurricane that led to widespread damage and destruction across many southern states during the summer of 2005. Areas impacted by the hurricane suffered widespread and extensive property damage, along with the adverse effects of the hurricane's storm surge and subsequent flooding. Hurricane Katrina has been identified as the third most intense hurricane impacting the United States, after the hurricanes that occurred in 1935 and 1969. The death toll from Hurricane Katrina from all causes totaled at least 1245, and property damage was estimated at more than $125 billion.[7]

The state of Mississippi suffered massive damage from the hurricane.[8] Especially extensive damage occurred to the communities located near where the eye wall passed over the communities of Waveland and Bay St. Louis. Data available from the National Weather Service indicated that as the hurricane passed over those communities, sustained winds of 120 mph occurred. The associated 27-foot storm surge led to near-total destruction of property and widespread flooding in these areas. In the immediate aftermath of the hurricane, first responders experienced significant difficulty gaining access to impacted communities, as well as the community of Gulfport, Mississippi. Access was complicated by debris, street and road destruction, flooding, and structural collapse, along with other barriers and impediments.

Federal Emergency Management Agency (FEMA) personnel responded to the area with several search and rescue teams. These search and rescue teams are part of the larger national urban search and rescue response system, which is made up of 28 specialized teams geographically spread across the United States.[9] Teams have been strategically located such that response to catastrophic disasters is more timely, effective, and efficient. These specialized search and rescue response teams are often identified as the first responders making initial contact with those in impacted communities. Team members are tasked with looking for, finding, and providing initial medical care to those in a disaster.

The author's personal experience as a responder in Mississippi documented that search and rescue teams encountered vulnerable individuals in a number of facilities that lacked any sort of comprehensive disaster or emergency management plan. Numerous published reports indicated that inpatient facilities, often those housing special needs populations, were adversely impacted. As search and rescue teams made their way through the debris-covered streets of several Mississippi coastal communities, they encountered individuals from various special needs populations, including those with mental health disorders. Due to the widespread structural destruction, individuals were taking shelter in a variety of makeshift structures—for example, large cardboard boxes, structures put together with debris, or abandoned/destroyed vehicles including automobiles. In one case, an individual was discovered taking shelter in a boat more than 500 yards from any existing waterway.

In both Louisiana and Mississippi, local leaders were criticized for lack of planning and preparedness.[10] This lack of planning and preparedness also extended to the private sector. Many of the facilities housing special needs populations were the subject of much debate, discussion, and, in some cases, legal and/or court proceedings.[11]

Individuals located by search and rescue teams had to first be medically assessed to determine if any emergency medical conditions existed. In the event that an emergency medical condition was discovered, plans had to be made to evacuate the individual to medical care as quickly as possible. Once it was determined that an emergency medical condition was not present, assessments were completed to determine which needs existed. In many cases, it was determined that individuals completely lacked any form of shelter or housing, food or water, and any form of communication. Local resources became available as time went on to evacuate these individuals and place them in shelters, facilities, or other forms of housing.

Many difficulties were encountered during the initial response. Search and rescue teams were often unable to locate family,[12] and individuals frequently had no form of identification. Individuals often were either unaware of or unable to communicate their medical history, including past medical and surgical history, current medications in dosages, and allergies to medications and pharmaceuticals. Some individuals were suffering from stress-related exacerbations of mental health disorders. Search and rescue and other first responder teams are not equipped or trained to deal with many of these conditions. Many healthcare facilities also are not equipped to deal with a surge of patients with acute complications related to previously existing mental health disorders.[13]

Summary Points

1. Natural disasters such as Hurricane Katrina may adversely impact health equity.
2. Vulnerable and special needs populations exist widely in communities and require special consideration during disaster planning.
3. Public health at every level must advocate for health equity in disasters.
4. Dedicated and purposeful disaster planning is necessary to ensure health equity in the disaster setting.

▶ Application of CEPH MPH Competencies

This case study addresses CEPH competency 15.

Competency 15: Evaluate Policies for Their Impact on Public Health and Health Equity

As the frequency and complexity of natural and human-made disasters have seemingly increased, the application of competencies has assumed new importance. The future public health workforce is an integral component in the assurance of health equity. The processes occurring at every level of government serve as drivers for policy development.

The Mississippi DMH's policy state disaster preparedness and response plan serves as an example of public health inclusive planning and policy development and further substantiates plans put into place to promote health equity. A primary example of the plan's focus on health equity can be found in its sections relating to sheltering in place during disasters. Notably, the policy identifies necessary components for effectiveness, which include facility requirements to isolate the structure from specific threats, staff knowledge, and organizational requirements specific to incident management and leadership. The plan also details when to make decisions on sheltering in place, identifies examples, and specifies that training and drills are essential for timely implementation. The Mississippi plan is complete with appropriate policy on initiation, situational factors, location factors, and resource factors.

It is encouraging to note the breadth and complexity of the plan from a health equity perspective. Lessons learned from the summer of 2005 were clearly influential in policy and plan development. Vulnerable populations—in this instance, the mental health community population—have been provided with an effective policy, carefully developed to lead toward health equity. In the case of the policy related to sheltering in place, this vulnerable population would remain safe, and would retain access to resources such as trained and equipped professionals, appropriate medications, and adequate shelter. The plan is broadly applicable across the entire state, and is available to both the public and private sectors.

The inclusion of public health professionals during disaster planning leads to both horizontal and vertical health equity. Communities, made up of many individuals with many different needs, are treated equally and assurances of the availability of resources exist for all and not simply for more resource-laden communities.

Vulnerable or special needs population also rely upon vertical equity. Due to actual gaps existing in vulnerable or special needs populations, public health must place added importance and specific emphasis on treating individuals according to their level of need.

It is essential that policies be evaluated for the impact they have, and that public health leaders evaluate policies in relation to a broad array of issues. Disasters, both natural and human-made, are no exceptions. Vulnerable and special needs populations are at increased risk of suffering from health inequity. Public health competencies are ideally applied to ensuring health equity during all phases of disaster response. These competencies include, and are not limited to, the following areas:

1. Analytic and assessment
2. Policy development/program planning
3. Cultural competency
4. Community dimensions of practice
5. Public health science
6. Financial planning and management
7. Leadership and systems thinking

Discussion Questions

1. Identify methods for policy evaluation by public health in disaster and emergency planning. How would these policies have better positioned communities for recovery in the Hurricane Katrina aftermath?
2. Discuss methods to ensure health equity in disaster and emergency planning. List these methods and specifically consider their application in the aftermath of Hurricane Katrina.
3. Discuss methods to raise awareness of health inequities among the first responder and emergency management communities. Where is the interface between public health systems and emergency medical systems?
4. How can health equity be assured in a disaster or catastrophe? Globally? Nationally? Locally?

References

1. Gitterman, A. (2014). *Handbook of social practice with vulnerable and resilient populations* (3rd ed.). New York, NY: Columbia University Press.
2. Bethel, J. W., Foreman, A. N., & Burke, S. C. (2011). Disaster preparedness among medically vulnerable populations. *American Journal of Preventative Medicine, 40*(6), 139–143.
3. Paton, D., & Johnston, D. (2017). *Disaster resilience: An integrated approach* (2nd ed.). Springfield, IL: Charles C. Thomas Publisher.
4. Waugh, W. L. (2015). *Living with hazards dealing with disasters: An introduction to emergency management* (1st ed.). London, UK: Routledge Taylor and Francis Group.
5. Berke, P., Smith, G., & Lyles, W. (2012). Planning for resiliency: Evaluation of state hazard mitigation plans under the Disaster Mitigation Act. *Natural Hazards Review, 13*(2), 139–149.
6. State of Mississippi, Department of Mental Health. (2012). State disaster preparedness and response plan. Retrieved from http://www.dmh.ms.gov/wp-content/uploads/2012/07/DMH-Disaster-Plan-July-2012-Final-Draft.pdf
7. Stephens, K. U. Sr., Grew, D., Chin, K., Kadetz, P., Greenough, P. G., Burkle, F. M. Jr., ... Franklin, E. R. (2007). Excess mortality in the aftermath of Hurricane Katrina: A preliminary report. *Disaster Medicine and Public Health Preparedness, 1*(1), 15–20.

8. Fritz, H. M., Blount, C., Sokoloski, R., Singleton, J., Fuggle, A., McAdoo, B. G., … Tate, B. (2007). Hurricane Katrina storm surge distribution and field observations on the Mississippi barrier islands. *Estuarine, Coastal and Shelf Science, 74*(1–2), 12–20.

9. U.S. Department of Homeland Security, Office of the Inspector General. (2006). A performance review of FEMA's disaster management activities in response to Hurricane Katrina. Retrieved from https://www.oig.dhs.gov/assets/Mgmt/OIG_06-32_Mar06.pdf

10. Sobel, R. S., & Leeson, P. T. (2006). Government's response to Hurricane Katrina: A *Public Choice* analysis. *Public Choice, 127*(1–2), 55–73.

11. Laditka, S. B., Laditka, J. N., Xirasagar, S., Cornman, C. B., Davis, C. B., & Richter, J. V. E. (2008). Providing shelter to nursing home evacuees in disasters: Lessons from Hurricane Katrina. *American Journal of Public Health, 98*(7), 1288–1293.

12. Pate, B. L. (2008). Identifying and tracking disaster victims: State of the art technology review. *Family and Community Health, 31*(1), 23–34.

13. Kessler, R. C., Galea, S., Gruber, M. J., Sampson, N. A., Ursano, R. J., & Wessely, S. (2008). Trends in mental illness and suicidality after Hurricane Katrina. *Molecular Psychiatry, 13*(1), 374–384.

Leadership

CHAPTER 16

Collaboration Among County Health Department Directors to Formulate Realistic Response Plans in the Event of Mosquito-Borne Zika Outbreaks

David M. Claborn, DrPH

▶ Background

Recent outbreaks of Zika virus disease in the United States, as well as the disturbing birth defects associated with the infection, have greatly increased interest in this re-emerging disease. Although the virus has been known for many years, public health workers thought until recently that it caused only mild symptoms. However, in recent years, the virus has spread through many parts of the world and has been linked to serious conditions, including Guillain-Barré syndrome and microcephaly.[1]

The primary means of virus transmission is the bite of an infected mosquito; thus, Zika virus disease is a vector-borne disease. In the Americas, the primary vector of Zika virus is a mosquito known as the yellow fever mosquito (*Aedes aegypti*), an insect that also spreads the agents of dengue and chikungunya. It is highly evolved to share a domestic environment with humans, adapting easily to the standing water around houses and urban areas. Typical aquatic habitats for the larvae include used tires and artificial containers.[1] Other mosquito species are proven Zika vectors as well. One particularly important species is the Asian tiger mosquito (*A. albopictus*), an invasive species that was introduced to Florida in the 1980s. Although this mosquito has become dominant in the eastern part of the United States, the dispersal of this and other invasive mosquito species is not well documented.

Zika virus disease emerged in the United States in 2014, though all of the initial cases appeared to have been associated with travel to endemic regions or with sexual transmission. This situation changed in 2015, when local vector-borne transmission was demonstrated in Florida. In 2017, mosquito-borne transmission also occurred in Texas. The vector in both instances was thought to be the yellow fever mosquito, though the Asian tiger mosquito also occurred in the vicinity of the outbreaks.[1]

▶ Case Study

In 2016, the Centers for Disease Control and Prevention (CDC) published a map of the United States with a theoretical range of the yellow fever mosquito, the primary vector of the Zika virus.[2] The range was based on a model utilizing variables of ambient temperatures, environmental conditions, historical occurrence data, and human travel patterns. That map depicted southern and western parts of Missouri as being within the probable range of the yellow fever mosquito and, therefore, at risk of vector-borne Zika disease. At the same time, the Missouri Department of Health and Senior Services (MDHSS) reported cases of Zika virus in the state, most of which were associated with travel to endemic countries.

An exhaustive survey of mosquitoes had not been done in Missouri in at least 75 years, if ever. The recent arrivals of two invasive mosquito species with vector potential and the lack of current information on mosquito fauna of the state helped convince public health officials of the necessity of an up-to-date mosquito survey for the state. In addition to the need for a current faunal survey, the MDHSS was concerned about the capacity of local health departments to respond to community demands for mosquito control in the event of an outbreak of vector-borne Zika virus disease. Most counties and cities had little expertise in mosquito control or vector-borne disease transmission, and even fewer had the required equipment. The extent of the deficit in capacity for response, however, was not well documented. In addition, the MDHSS wanted to provide a standardized response plan that realistically reflected the capabilities of the local public health agencies, yet provided a list of effective responses that most of the counties and cities could implement.

The MDHSS contracted Missouri State University (MSU) in Springfield, Missouri, to conduct the faunal survey; to assess the local capacities for vector surveillance and control; to formulate an emergency vector control response plan; and to train local agencies on the implementation of that plan. This case study describes the process used to achieve these goals.

Case Study Phases

■ Phase 1: Intensive survey of vector fauna of Missouri.
■ Phase 2: Online survey of stakeholders as related to knowledge, capacity, and needs.
■ Phase 3: Formulation of realistic response measures by county health departments.
■ Phase 4: Training on response measures and how to formulate an emergency plan.

Phase 1: The Survey

In 2016 and 2017, researchers with MSU found surveillance sites in auto salvage yards and used-tire shops in urban or suburban areas throughout southern and western Missouri. Field workers used a variety of traps and baits to survey adult and larval mosquitoes on these sites. The survey workers trapped and identified more than 35,000 mosquitoes during the two-year survey. A total of 31 different species were identified. Contrary to what the CDC model suggested, the survey failed to detect the presence of the yellow fever mosquito. The same was not true of the secondary vector, the Asian tiger mosquito. This invasive species had been reported in Missouri previously, but its abundance and distribution were not known prior to the survey. It turned out to be very abundant and present in all 31 counties in which the survey occurred. Another invasive species with potential as a vector, the Asian bush mosquito (*A. japonicus*), was also widespread across the state.

The conclusion of the survey was that there was an abundant population of potential Zika vectors in Missouri, such that the transmission of the virus in the state was at least theoretically possible. However, the survey demonstrated that the majority of mosquitoes in the region were Asian tiger mosquitoes.

Phase 2: Assessment of Knowledge and Needs of Stakeholders

In 2016, the MDHSS Section for Disease Prevention hosted a statewide meeting of county health departments to share information and to encourage collaboration on a variety of public health issues. The Section decided to use this meeting as a forum through which to find public health workers with concerns about the risk of Zika transmission in their jurisdictions, especially those who might be responsible for public health efforts in the wake of a mosquito-borne outbreak of the disease. The MDHSS considered these persons to be the primary stakeholders with regard to this issue.

The MSU researchers gave one presentation on the mosquito survey at a general session as part of the effort to recruit stakeholders, then followed up at the same workshop with two "listening sessions" in which the researchers recorded concerns, perceptions, and questions of the stakeholders. The researchers also used direct questioning of the stakeholders to assess levels of education and the local capacity for performing vector surveillance and control. In addition, all stakeholders were provided with an opportunity to complete a more extensive written survey that addressed these same issues.

TABLE 16-1 Themes from Stakeholders at Planning Conference Concerning Emergency Vector Control in the Event of Local Zika Transmission

- "It is important to have a common message across all jurisdictions in the state."

- "The message should be measured and appropriate without exaggeration."

- "Use good data to put the message into perspective."

- "We need legal guidance. What is the law regarding our responsibilities and what we can do?"

- "Mapping of larval sites can occur while doing day-to-day business."

- "Sanitation efforts could use volunteers like the adopt-a-highway program."

- "The state should consider raising the tire disposal fee from 50 cents to 1 dollar, with the additional funds going into vector control."

- "There is no vector control capacity in most counties and cities. The only options in these areas are public education and counseling of infected persons."

In addition to the quantitative data from the written survey, stakeholders in attendance were encouraged to provide unstructured comments about their needs with regard to planning for possible disease transmission in their counties.[3] Qualitative themes from these comments are summarized in **TABLE 16-1**.

From the survey and the listening sessions, it became obvious that the counties were not funded to respond to an outbreak of any vector-borne disease, including Zika. In addition, most counties had no personnel with adequate background and experience to perform standard mosquito surveillance and control activities. One specific comment, however, seemed to provide a potential way forward. One stakeholder stated that it would be possible to map larval development sites such as wrecking yards and piles of used tires while engaged in other business of the county health department. This statement was discussed further at the conference, and most county directors agreed that such mapping was possible. This consensus was to serve as the eventual basis for recommendations to counties regarding plans in the event of local mosquito-borne transmission.

Phase 3: Response Plan

The information from the county directors and other stakeholders led to several conclusions, as noted in **TABLE 16-2**.

In discussions between the MSU researchers and the MDHSS leadership, it became obvious that any efforts in this arena would have to be accomplished with little extra investment of money or staffing. The mosquito survey, however, did suggest that the vast majority of mosquitoes developing in artificial containers in the

TABLE 16-2 Conclusions About County Capabilities and Needs

1. Counties and cities are not sufficiently funded or staffed to be able to plan for or respond to an outbreak of mosquito-borne Zika virus disease.

2. Few counties have the expertise required to do the recommended surveillance and control efforts.

3. Current funding and manning levels are unlikely to change favorably in the near future.

4. Most public health workers do not think the likelihood of a vector-borne outbreak is high enough to justify diversion of current funds and personnel toward addressing the issue.

5. Efforts to plan and prepare for such an outbreak that can be done while accomplishing routine tasks should be carried out, but the relatively low risk of an outbreak does not justify large investments in training or equipment.

state were the Asian tiger mosquito, a secondary vector of the Zika virus; the other mosquitoes occurred in much smaller numbers. Based on this observation, the MSU researchers recommended that public health agencies assume that any mosquito larvae or pupae detected in an artificial container were Asian tiger mosquitoes. Making this simplification allowed the county health directors to eliminate the need for specialized training. Techniques to survey mosquitoes are easy to master as long as they do not have to be identified to genus or species.

By mapping places where any mosquito larvae occurred in artificial containers, the county health departments could come up with a plan for emergency mosquito control in the event of a disease outbreak. The plan would consist of mapping areas with large numbers of artificial containers in which mosquitoes were present and that were near human populations, then identifying local resources that could be contracted to effect mosquito control in the event of a disease outbreak. Such a plan required little extra effort and no expertise beyond that currently in the county departments. Based on these conclusions, the counties could build a realistic and useful response plan without substantial investment in money or personnel. It should be noted that the assumptions of this plan were possible only because the mosquito survey showed that the Asian tiger mosquito accounted for nearly 70% of the mosquitoes surveyed in artificial containers.

Phase 4: Training

In the summer of 2018, the MDHSS and MSU researchers held three meetings around the state to train approximately 120 county public health workers on how to construct a simplified response plan based on the results of the statewide vector survey.

Summary Points

1. Stakeholders at county health departments stated they had no expertise or staffing to effect mosquito surveillance or to plan for vector-borne disease outbreaks.
2. A statewide survey demonstrated that most mosquitoes were of one species, so local surveys could be simplified by assuming larval mosquitoes were of the dominant species.
3. The MDHSS trained county representatives to use a simplified survey technique to map areas with high mosquito populations and to make emergency response plans in the event of a disease outbreak.

▶ Application of CEPH MPH Competencies

This case study addresses CEPH competencies 16 and 13.

Competency 16: Apply Principles of Leadership, Governance, and Management, Which Include Creating a Vision, Empowering Others, Fostering Collaboration, and Guiding Decision Making

Stakeholders agreed that simplified surveillance based on the findings of the state-wide mosquito survey could be accomplished while performing other required tasks as part of the counties' public health responsibilities. Although not ideal, this simplification allowed county public health workers to formulate realistic county response plans based on mapping of high-risk areas and identification of mosquito control resources in the event they were required.

These early stages of the planning process served to bring together several persons who were stakeholders in the issue of vector-borne Zika virus disease, including state health workers, county health department directors, and academic researchers. These stakeholders rapidly formulated a goal of constructing plans for reasonable responses to increased disease risk in the absence of technical expertise or increased funding. This was achieved primarily by identifying the primary stakeholders early in the process and providing a forum in which they could share concerns, identify needs and assets, and then formulate a vision and objectives for a way forward. U.S. President Dwight Eisenhower once reportedly said, "The plan is nothing; planning is everything." Perhaps providing a forum in which stakeholders meet to formulate a common vision and identify potential collaborative efforts is one of the most important parts of public health planning.

Competency 13: Propose Strategies to Identify Stakeholders and Build Coalitions and Partnerships for Influencing Public Health Outcomes

Early in the project, the MDHHS made the decision to define stakeholders as public health workers who would be responsible for any decisions or efforts to control Zika virus disease in the event of a local outbreak of mosquito-borne disease. This decision allowed facilitators to conduct inclusive discussions that accurately identified local capacities to respond to outbreaks. The discussions revolved around a vision of a realistic and collaborative plan to respond to potential outbreaks in the absence of increased funding or staffing.

Discussion Questions

1. Why was the input from stakeholders important in formulating realistic response plans for this situation?
2. Were other stakeholders excluded from this process? If so, who?
3. How could the process of identifying stakeholders be improved?

References

1. Moreno-Madrinan, M. J., & Turrell, M. (2018). History of mosquito-borne diseases in the United States and implications for new pathogens. *Emerging Infectious Diseases, 24*(5), 821–826.
2. Centers for Disease Control and Prevention. (2017, September). Surveillance and control of *Aedes aegypti* and *Aedes albopictus* in the United States. Retrieved from https://www.cdc.gov /chikungunya/resources/vector-control.html
3. Claborn, D. M., Thompson, K. R., & Duitsman, D. (2017). *Planning document for Missouri Surveillance and Control Action Plan*. Ozark Public Health Institute Report. Springfield, MO: Missouri State University.

CHAPTER 17

Flint Water Case Study: Negotiation and Mediation

Laura Erskine, PhD, MBA

▶ Background

The Safe Drinking Water Act (SWDA) is a federal law to regulate drinking water in the United States. Under the SWDA, the U.S. Environmental Protection Agency (EPA) can create regulations if any identified contaminant is known to occur in public water systems often enough, or at levels high enough, to cause a public health concern.[1] The EPA regulates potential contaminants through the National Primary Drinking Water Regulations (NPDWR).[2]

Some contaminants, including lead, result from corroding water pipes. All large systems (serving communities of more than 50,000 residents) were required to have corrosion control measures in place by 1997.[3] To prevent corrosion, water managers add orthophosphate to their municipal water supplies.[4] The orthophosphate bonds with lead in the pipes, preventing any chemical interaction between the lead and water. However, unless the orthophosphate is added continually, the barrier breaks down, and lead leaches into the water flowing through the pipes. The Flint River water had high levels of chloride, which accelerates corrosion. In addition to naturally occurring chloride, two possible sources for the high levels of chloride in the Flint River were ferric chloride used in conjunction with chlorine disinfection and dissolved road salt applied to manage snow and ice during Michigan winters.[4]

Exposure to lead can be extremely dangerous. In children, all organs are susceptible to lead poisoning, and adverse effects can be seen in the form of damage to the brain and nervous system, slowed growth and development, hearing and speech problems, and learning and behavior problems. Any of these can lower a child's IQ, decrease the child's ability to pay attention, and cause underperformance in school. In adults, lead poisoning can result in anemia, high blood pressure, balance problems, altered hormone levels, and kidney problems.[5,6] Most symptoms do not reveal themselves until many years after the initial exposure.[7]

One of the most concerning aspects of lead exposure is that once it has been deposited in the nervous system, lead cannot be removed. The impact of lead poisoning on neurological development is permanent. Recent research has indicated that, with each 1 microgram per deciliter increase in blood lead level, children demonstrate decreasing performance on intelligence tests.[8]

In a letter published in *Health Affairs*, Peter Muennig shared analysis showing that the lifelong bill for individual lead exposure incidents is $50,000 and 0.2 year of perfect health. In Flint, there were more than 8,000 individual exposures ($400 million) and 1,760 adjusted life-years lost.[9]

▶ Case Study[8,10,11]

Flint, Michigan, is a majority Black city where approximately 40% of residents live in poverty. The size of the population plunged from 200,000 residents in 1960 to a little more than 100,000 in 2011, and the combination of poverty and a shrinking population led to a financial crisis. In Michigan, when a city is under severe financial stress, the state can appoint an Emergency Manager with broad power to make decisions. One of the cost-cutting measures explored by Flint Emergency Manager Ed Kurtz and other city officials was a search for less expensive water. By ending the city's contract with the Detroit Water and Sewage Department (DWSD) and joining the Karegnondi Water Authority (KWA), officials expected to save $5 million for the city of Flint. However, on April 25, 2014, the official switch was made instead to the Flint River because the pipeline connecting Flint to KWA was not yet operational. While state and local officials internally predicted problems, a press release announced the water "safe to drink."

Complaints from residents started in May 2014. People had problems with both the smell and the color of the water. In September 2014, Flint violated the SDWA for the first time. By October 2014, the local General Motors plant had switched the source of its water because corrosion was found on brand-new equipment. Complaints from local residents (mainly from low-income people of color) continued to be ignored by local and state officials.

Flint was found in violation of the SDWA for a second time in January 2015, when disinfection by-products (resulting from the interaction between chlorine and organic matter in the water) were discovered. While some types of disinfection by-products are possible carcinogens in humans, Flint officials maintained no emergency was occurring and stated they were seeking a solution that would resolve the problem. Simultaneously, state government offices supplied employees based in Flint with bottled water.

LeeAnn Walters, a Flint resident, demanded tests of lead levels in the water in her home in February 2015. City tests revealed elevated lead levels (104 parts per billion) that exceeded the 15 ppb limit employed by the EPA. Walters subsequently reported that her children had been diagnosed with lead poisoning, and she sent 100 water samples to a research team at Virginia Tech University. These independent tests by a research team at Virginia Tech University showed lead levels as high at 13,200 ppb. The EPA designates water as hazardous waste when lead levels reach 5,000 ppb. The Michigan Department of Environmental Quality

(MDEQ) also reported to the EPA that Flint did not implement the required corrosion controls. The American Civil Liberties Union (ACLU) picked up a leaked EPA memo expressing concern about lead levels but a MDEQ spokesperson said publicly, "anyone who is concerned about lead in the drinking water in Flint can relax."

By the fall of 2015, the Virginia Tech research team had expanded the water testing to hundreds of homes in Flint. The researchers reported lead levels to be among the worst the team had seen in decades, while city and state officials questioned the results and suggested that the team found elevated lead levels only because the researchers wanted to support their hypothesis. At the same time, Mona Hanna Attisha and doctors at Hurley Medical Center in Flint took the surprising step of holding a press conference to release data showing that the percentage of children younger than 5 years old with elevated lead levels had doubled throughout Flint and almost tripled in the inner city. While officials at the Michigan Department of Public Health and Human Services blamed elevated lead results on seasonal changes, two experts summarized the adverse effects of lead:

> Lead is a devastating poison. It damages children's brains, erodes intelligence, diminishes creativity and the ability to weigh consequences and make good decisions, impairs language skills, shortens attention span, and predisposes to hyperactive and aggressive behavior. Lead exposure in early childhood is linked to later increased risk for dyslexia and school failure.[12]

Finally, officials acted and Governor Snyder announced a plan to provide free water filters and additional testing in October 2015. The city of Flint also switched back to the Detroit water supply (now called Great Lakes Water Authority). After Karen Weaver beat Flint mayor Dayne Walling in a November election, she declared a state of emergency for the city. That same month, the Flint Water Advisory Task Force (created by the governor) released a preliminary report placing blame on the MDEQ, and two MDEQ officials resigned. In January 2015, Hilary Clinton raised the issue during her presidential campaigning, and Governor Rick Snyder, President Barack Obama, and the EPA all declared a state of emergency. The Federal Emergency Management Agency (FEMA) was then authorized to provide water, water filters, and other equipment to the area, and a Medicaid Section 1115 waiver submitted by Governor Snyder was expedited and approved by the Centers for Medicare and Medicaid Services (CMS). The waiver expanded Medicaid and Children's Health Insurance Program (CHIP) eligibility, waived cost-sharing and premiums for Flint beneficiaries, and expanded Medicaid Targeted Case Management to coordinate support services for all Medicaid-eligible children and pregnant women.

Between April and July 2016, criminal charges were filed against 15 individuals involved in the scandal, ranging from willful neglect of duty to involuntary manslaughter. Rather than paying the equivalent of $100/day to treat the corrosive pipes, Flint is now responsible for the $1.5 billion required to fix Flint's water problems (**FIGURE 17-1**). Sadly, most residents have lost so much trust in government that they are unlikely to drink tap water as long as they remain in Flint. People are suffering from both mental and physical ailments as a result of lead poisoning, and some (including activists from Flint Rising) are calling for all Flint residents to receive fully subsidized health care.

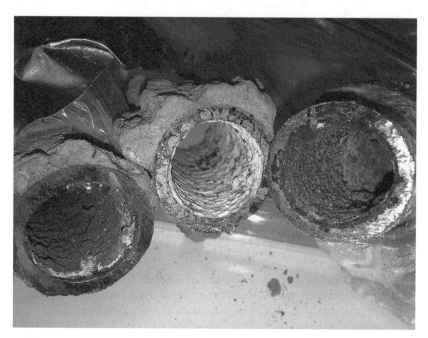

FIGURE 17-1 Damaged pipes.

Courtesy of Marc Edwards.

Summary Points[13]

1. The switch to the Flint River as a municipal water source caused water distribution pipes to corrode and leach lead and other contaminants into local drinking water.
2. Officials failed to respond to resident complaints for more than a year and questioned the legitimacy of outside data analysis when it was made public.
3. Officials did not disclose internal concerns about the adequacy of the distribution pipes, the lack of corrosion treatment processes, or internal data about elevated lead levels.
4. In October 2016, Flint residents were advised to drink local tap water only if it had been filtered through an approved filter certified to remove lead.
5. In addition to the negative health effects from lead exposure, there are ongoing concerns about the behavioral health of Flint residents.

▶ Application of CEPH MPH Competencies

This case study addresses CEPH competency 17.

Competency 17: Apply Negotiation and Mediation Skills to Address Organizational or Community Challenges

Public health, healthcare delivery, and healthcare policy are currently in a state of flux. Negotiation and mediation are important tools to work through the uncertainty that accompanies change. In addition, the context is one in which different parties can have different interests and different ideas about how to develop innovative solutions. There are tensions between prevention and treatment, tensions around costs and payments, anxiety caused by uncertainty and lack of transparency, and fundamental questions about the role of the public sector.

To apply negotiation and mediation skills, students need to understand these concepts more fully. Negotiation is an interpersonal decision-making process used when single parties cannot reach their objectives singlehandedly.[14] The challenge for negotiators is that they often have some objectives and goals that are shared and others that are at odds with each other. Members of the Harvard Negotiation Project developed the Seven Elements framework to describe the essential tools required for successful negotiation.[15]

1. Interests are our basic needs, wants, and motivations. These are rarely shared openly, but are such an important guide for what we do that experienced negotiators will work hard to determine the underlying interests behind the stated positions of the other party.

2. Legitimacy and fairness are critical to successful negotiating. People will often reject an offer they perceive as unfair, even if it would leave them objectively better off.

3. Relationships are especially important when parties will continue to interact. It can be very beneficial to take some time to build a strong relationship between negotiation partners by demonstrating high ethical and personal standards.

4. Negotiation preparation must include an analysis of your Best Alternative to a Negotiated Agreement (BATNA). Alternatives give each party positions to fall back on if the negotiation does not work out.

5. Options (including conditions, contingencies, and trades) refer to available choices that parties might consider to bridge differences.

6. When negotiating, a commitment is akin to a promise and can range from a verbal agreement to a signed contract.

7. Communication choices can drive the success or failure. These choices can include the channel, tone and language, and whether the parties brainstorm jointly or present demands.

In addition to the strategic and tactical elements described in the Seven Elements, the role of emotion is very important. Research shows that anger can lead to extremely poor outcomes by escalating conflict, biasing perceptions, and making impasses more likely. Anger damages relationships and makes future negotiations unproductive. Anxiety can result in suboptimal outcomes, as people experiencing anxiety make weaker first offers and are more likely to exit early.[16]

When negotiators reach an impasse or the level of conflict is too high, it may be time to call for a mediator. A mediator is a third party trained in negotiation and conflict resolution who can help parties reach a mutual agreement. Mediators attempt to alter the negotiators' behaviors and to improve their behaviors toward each other. This can often be more complex than the challenges faced by the negotiators themselves.[17] There are three basic styles of mediation, ordered here from most passive to most assertive: facilitative, formulative, and manipulative.[15] Across the spectrum, mediation is successful in approximately 60% of cases.

Discussion Questions

There are several groups with different interests in this case: government entities (MDEQ, MDHHS, Michigan governor's office, state-appointed emergency managers, City of Flint officials, Genesee County Health Department, U.S. EPA, CMS), local residents (LeeAnn Walters, Melissa Mays, Angela McIntosh), activist and advocacy groups (American Civil Liberties Union, unions, Flint Rising, Concerned Pastors for Social Action, Rainbow PUSH Coalition, Greater Flint Health Coalition, Food & Water Watch), researchers and technical experts (Virginia Tech Water Study Team), doctors (Mona Hanna-Attisha, Lawrence Reynolds), and media (MLive, Detroit Free Press, NPR).

1. Identify missed opportunities for negotiation and/or mediation both before the water source was changed to the Flint River and in the years since then.
2. Role-play the different actors/groups to create a plan for moving forward. Be faithful to the interests and positions of the respective parties. Ensure that the plan is culturally sensitive, financially feasible, and works to restore trust.
3. Should requirements for mediation be written into public health regulations? Why or why not? If so, how could that be implemented?

References

1. Environmental Protection Agency. (2017, May 22). Drinking water contaminants: Standards and regulations. Retrieved from https://www.epa.gov/dwstandardsregulations
2. National Primary Drinking Water Regulations, 40 C.F.R. pt 141 (2007).
3. Lead and copper rule: A quick reference guide. (2008). Retrieved from https://nepis.epa.gov/Exe/ZyPDF.cgi?Dockey=60001N8P.txt
4. Augenbraun, E., & Chain, L. (Producers). (2016, February 25). Corrosive chemistry: How lead ended up in Flint's drinking water [Video file]. Retrieved from https://www.scientificamerican.com/video/corrosive-chemistry-how-lead-ended-up-in-flint-s-drinking-water1/
5. Centers for Disease Control and Prevention. (2018, May 4). Lead. Retrieved from https://www.cdc.gov/nceh/lead/
6. Murata, K., Iwata, T., Dakeishi, M., & Karita, K. (2009). Lead toxicity: Does the critical level of lead resulting in adverse effects differ between adults and children? *Journal of Occupational Health, 51* (1), 1–12. doi:10.1539/joh.k8003
7. Campbell, C., Greenberg, R., Mankikar, D., & Ross, R. (2016). A case study of environmental injustice: The failure in Flint. *International Journal of Environmental Research and Public Health, 13* (10), 951. doi:10.3390/ijerph13100951
8. Davis, M. M., Kolb, C., Rothstein, E., Reynolds, L., & Sikkema, K. (2016). *Flint Water Advisory Task Force final report.* Retrieved from https://www.michigan.gov/documents/snyder/FWATF_FINAL_REPORT_21March2016_517805_7.pdf
9. Muennig, P. (2016). The social costs of lead poisonings. *Health Affairs, 35* (8), 1545–1545. doi:10.1377/hlthaff.2016.0661
10. Michigan Radio. (n.d.). Not safe to drink. Retrieved from http://michiganradio.org/topic/not-safe-drink
11. Longley, K. (2012, December 1). Flint emergency: Timeline of state takeover (with photo gallery). Retrieved from http://www.mlive.com/news/flint/index.ssf/2012/12/flint_emergency_timeline_of_st_1.html
12. Landrigan, P., & Bellinger, D. (2016, April 11). How to finally end lead poisoning in America. Retrieved from http://time.com/4286726/lead-poisoning-in-america/
13. Centers for Disease Control and Prevention, National Center for Environmental Health, Division of Environmental Hazards and Health Effects, Health Studies Branch. (2016). *Community Assessment for Public Health Emergency Response (CASPER) after the Flint water*

crisis: *May 17–19, 2016.* Retrieved from https://www.cdc.gov/nceh/hsb/disaster/casper /docs/Flint_MI_CASPER_Report_508.pdf

14. Thompson, L. L. (2015). *The mind and heart of the negotiator.* London, UK: Pearson.
15. Moffitt, M. L., & Bordone, R. C. (2005). *The handbook of dispute resolution.* San Francisco, CA: Jossey-Bass.
16. Brooks, A. W. (2015, December). Emotion and the art of negotiation. *Harvard Business Review,* 56–64.
17. Druckman, D., & Wall, J. A. (2017). A treasure trove of insights. *Journal of Conflict Resolution, 61* (9), 1898–1924. doi:10.1177/0022002717721388

Communication

CHAPTER 18

Interagency Communication and Public Information During Disasters and Emergencies

Angela G. Clendenin, PhD, MA

▶ Background

Disasters and emergencies create chaotic communications environments. This chaos is full of "mental noise" or distractions precluding full attention to messaging.[1] It is during this time, when the importance of information and the impact of distractions are both increased, that individuals have a reduced capacity to remember the information they receive. In fact, it is estimated that people in crisis mode retain only about 20% of the information with which they are provided.[2]

However, failure to effectively communicate during a disaster is costly not only in terms of rescue operations but also in increased rates of morbidity and mortality.[3] Trying to process critical, rapidly disseminated, and complex information in a disaster/emergency environment oftentimes results in conflicting information, decreased self-efficacy, and significant costs of response and rescue operations (not including loss of life).[3,4] Post-hurricane analysis after Hurricane Ike hit the coast of Texas in 2008 determined the failure to follow official evacuation orders increased rescue operation costs by nearly 2000%. Similarly, 4 years after the 2011 tsunami and subsequent nuclear reactor meltdown in Fukushima, Japan, thousands of Japanese citizens now note increased mistrust of authority after mixed, conflicting messages disseminated by the government forced people to be evacuated into contaminated areas twice before they arrived at a safe location.[4]

Risk and crisis communication are very similar concepts, which may be defined as "the effort by concerned experts to provide information to allow an individual, stakeholder, or an entire community to make the best possible decisions about their well-being within nearly impossible time constraints and help people ultimately to accept the imperfect nature of choices during the crisis."[5] Currently, evidence-based practices for risk and crisis communication include a focus on being concise by limiting the number of key messages for dissemination and ensuring the timely release of consistent information.[6-9] Such messages may include information on sheltering in place, curfews, infection control, and evacuation routes. Research has shown individuals will believe in and follow such guidance when the person or entity delivering the information is deemed trustworthy.[10] Trustworthiness, however, is a complex construct encompassing both perceived empathy and expertise.[11] However, expertise is now proving to be a complex concept in and of itself, with individual experiences and perceptions leading to different denotative and connotative definitions of expertise even within seemingly homogenous populations.[12] In its current state, then, risk and crisis communication is an inherently complicated practice, despite decades of research into evidence-based guidance and training, consisting of multiple moving parts.

Training for those responsible for sharing information with the public in times of emergencies and disasters is offered through state and federal emergency management agencies such as the Texas Division of Emergency Management and the Federal Emergency Management Agency (FEMA). These courses emphasize the importance of a consistent message disseminated through a unified response structure.[13] However, different emergency response organizations often have different information that needs to reach different targeted audiences, as well as different resources and capacity. In addition, the relationships established between such response agencies and the public outside of emergencies and disasters may often lead to individuals seeking information from one organization when another has stepped in during an emergency to take the lead in a given area. This indicates the important need for agencies to think more broadly about going beyond just a consistent message—that is, to develop interagency communication processes that build a flexible foundation enabling them to easily guide the public to the information and resources they need on what could potentially be the worst day of their lives.

▶ Case Study

On August 25, 2017, Hurricane Harvey hit the Texas coast as a Category 4 hurricane with sustained winds of close to 130 mph, nearly 27 trillion gallons of water falling over Texas and parts of Louisiana, and 33 Texas counties under federal disaster declaration.[14,15] More than 31,000 federal employees were joined by a similar number of state employees and more than 300,000 volunteers from nongovernmental organizations (NGOs) to assist in the response effort.[16] The challenges faced by these responding agencies and organizations included how to ensure people who needed assistance were connected with those who had resources to provide the assistance. As of November 30, 2017, approximately $31 billion had been spent or committed for Harvey relief and recovery efforts.[17]

A large portion of the response effort involved a significant number of rescues of both animals and people by responders entering into hazardous conditions.

By September 22, 2017, it was estimated more than 122,000 rescues had been conducted.[18] Both rescuers and the rescued alike faced significant public health risks.

Storm surge from the coast brought copious amounts of saltwater inland, contaminating sources of freshwater. The U.S. Department of Agriculture reported a significant number of unevaluated animals were at high risk of salt toxicity from the remaining brackish water.[19] In addition, much of the floodwater entering the drinking water supply was reported to be contaminated with sewage and chemicals, many of which are known to be extremely toxic to humans and animals.[20,21] The extreme heat and humidity created ideal conditions for explosive growth of mold and bacteria. Indeed, public health officials regularly reported worrisome daily coliform counts, as well as an increasing number of deaths and injuries due to drowning, electrocutions from downed powerlines, and asphyxiation due to carbon monoxide poising (from using generators in closed environments).

Another long-term public health concern resulting from Hurricane Harvey was the increased risk from mosquito-borne disease. The Texas Department of State Health Services (DSHS) reported that, in addition to 990 medical response missions, 3200 medical patient evacuations, 1800 patients treated by mobile medical units, and 70,000 vaccinations provided, 6,765,971 acres were treated for mosquito control as a preventive action against infectious diseases such as West Nile virus, Zika, and chikungunya.[22] Anecdotal evidence also arose regarding rashes and skin conditions from exposure to contaminated floodwater.

The Challenges of Communication

With information about evacuations, food safety, illness and injury prevention, assistance with resources, resource donation, and hazard risks all needing to be communicated to a diverse audience of government officials, responding organizations, and the public, there was a significant challenge in coordinating messages across multiple agencies focused on their specific area of response and across large distances. How do you inform people, who are already in a crisis state, about the health risks they face from mosquitoes, mold, mildew, bacteria- and toxin-laden water, food safety, and other environmental hazards without creating confusing messages? How do you connect people in need with those who can provide? How do you place more than 30,000 responders on the same page between the public in need and those responsible for guiding the response effort?

Indeed, it has been noted that "when disaster strikes, [this] complex task environment requires multiple organization to transform from autonomous actors into interdependent decision-making teams . . . [and] the ability to provide quality and timeliness of information shapes the effectiveness of emergency response efforts."[23] Because of the fluid, ever-changing nature of disaster response, it is common for response agencies to focus on their specific mission. As an agency is often required to spread out its resources, elements from within the same agency may find themselves operating in a disconnect from the larger whole. This necessitates a need to communicate internally as well as across agency "lanes."

Based on phone calls and social media inquiries during Hurricane Harvey, it was evident that people were seeking places to evacuate to with their animals (including livestock) and needed supplies both for their animals and for their families, and that others had those resources to offer. The question became how to facilitate the connection between these groups. If each agency just responded to the inquiries it received, many connections would have been missed. In addition, as the rain dissipated, leaving standing water and high humidity in many places, impacted residents began to express concerns about mold, mosquitoes, and "muddy" water.

The decision was made to include all animal response agencies (Texas A&M Veterinary Emergency Team, Texas Animal Health Commission, sheltering partners, Texas A&M AgriLife Extension) and the DSHS in a once-daily (twice-daily, if needed) phone conference to evaluate requests. As an outgrowth of these phone calls, the creation of #HarveyHotline, a phone number and corresponding social media hashtag, enabled all agencies to consistently steer those in need of information or items to one central location so they could be connected with those who had information to provide. The Harvey Hotline was included in every agency's social media presence, in traditional media interviews, and across both animal and human internal agency communications. The spanning of these boundaries ensured information and resources were shared with a broader spectrum of the public, both urban and rural, in a consistent and efficient manner. Given the diversity of the area hit by Hurricane Harvey, the ability to recognize and respond to the differing needs of the people impacted facilitated a more unified step toward recovery. Using multiple platforms to create essentially a "net," each agency not only reached its specific audience but also those tuned in to other agencies.

Summary Points

1. Large-scale disasters involve multiple response agencies and a diverse public with differing needs.
2. During a crisis, reaching an increased number of people requires cooperation and collaboration.
3. Response agencies are often faced with the challenges of limited resources and a focus on agency-centric missions.
4. A scheme to span boundaries and connect agencies together extends the reach of all agencies.

▶ Application of CEPH MPH Competencies

This case study addresses CEPH competencies 18 and 17.

Competency 18: Select Communication Strategies for Different Audiences and Sectors

Hurricane Harvey proved to be challenging for response efforts. As mentioned earlier, it was an unprecedented storm requiring unprecedented communication strategies. In the past, multiple agencies were able to disseminate messages crafted for their specific audiences with minimal cross-coordination. In the case of Harvey, however, the overwhelming need to provide aid and the numerous requests for help and guidance quickly overwhelmed the previous strategies used in prior disasters. The population impacted by Harvey was diverse, including both urban and rural residents living in areas of both high and low socioeconomic status. There were pet owners, livestock owners, and those who owned both. In addition, multiple languages are spoken along the Texas coast, with differing cultural values determining whether people responded through evacuation or sheltering in place.

For the residents in need to be able to quickly understand the public health hazards from the standing water and downed powerlines, find available resources to move out of harm's way, and prepare for recovery by comprehending simple concepts such as food and drinking water safety concerns after a disaster required a multi-agency communication response. Each agency, by sharing information on a daily basis, were then able to disseminate the necessary information through media (both social and traditional) in a manner appropriate to those needing the guidance. Not every resident places trust in every agency, and certainly not every person sought information from the multiple agencies involved in the Harvey-impacted areas. Being able to turn to trusted sources and get a consistent message assured residents they could place confidence in what was being said.

One example of how this "net" had a positive impact on the communities hard hit by Harvey involved the explanation of mosquito control concerns. Even though the actual spokespeople at each agency were not environmental scientists, epidemiologists, or entomologists, gathering information from the DSHS surveillance experts helped all agencies communicate the dangers of an exploding mosquito population post Harvey, as well as explain how residents could protect themselves and their pets from both the mosquitoes and the spraying conducted to eradicate as many of the disease vectors as possible. The agencies' dissemination of agency-specific information tagged with the Harvey Hotline number enabled many residents to access a preferred source and then receive information they perhaps would not have received otherwise.

Competency 17: Apply Negotiation and Mediation Skills to Address Organizational or Community Challenges

This case was also a demonstration of leadership. With so many agencies having so much information to disseminate, each thinking its own message was most important, negotiation and mediation became a necessity to provide the organizational foundation for consistent communication. It was decided that a state agency, the Texas Animal Health Commission, had the best linkages to people in the impacted area, as well as the capacity to create and manage a hotline. This organization became the hub of the "net" created and established the daily teleconferences. All the other agencies attended the conferences, shared information gathered from the field, discussed important guidance to be disseminated, and invited in other agencies as the environment and response effort changed over time.

It has been shown previously that effective and timely communication can save lives in a disaster. Moreover, the bigger the disaster, the more necessary it becomes, as an agency spokesperson, to act as a boundary-spanner and connect the agency and the agency's audience with a broader source of information. This creates a solid foundation of confidence upon which people in need can base their protective action decisions, and it empowers them to do so from an informed perspective.

Discussion Questions

1. The agencies listed in this case study were predominantly animal related, with the exception of the Texas Department of State Health Services. Which

other groups might have benefited from participating in the Harvey Hotline effort, and why?

2. Within just the public health realm, a number of messages needed to be pushed out in the hurricane's aftermath: food safety after loss of electricity, flooded roadways, generator use, mosquito risks, bacteria and toxins in the water, and so on. How would you begin to prioritize these messages without overwhelming the public by pushing them out all at once?

3. Understanding communication and demonstrating leadership are fundamental core competencies for public health graduates. Are there other disaster- or emergency-specific competencies (e.g., personal preparedness) that are also important to ensuring a prepared public health workforce? If so, what might these be?

4. Some sources suggest a best practice is constant communication with the public, even in between disasters. How might this have a negative impact on communication once a disaster strikes?

References

1. Covello, V. T. (2011). Risk communication, radiation, and radiological emergencies: Strategies, tools, and techniques. *Health Physics, 101*(5), 511–530.

2. Covello, V. T., Minamyer, S., & Clayton, K. (2007). *Effective risk and crisis communication during water security emergencies.* New York, NY: National Homeland Security Center.

3. Dorell, O. (2008, September 15). Almost 2,000 Ike survivors rescued. *USA Today.* Retrieved from http://usatoday30.usatoday.com/weather/hurricane/2008-09-14-ike-main_N.htm

4. *World Nuclear News.* (2012). Fukushima evacuees failed by information flow. Retrieved from http://www.world-nuclear-news.org/RS-Fukushima_evacuees_failed_by_information_flow -1206127.html

5. Quinn, S. C., & Reynolds, B. (2008). Effective communication during an influenza pandemic: The value of using a crisis and emergency risk communication framework. *Health Promotion Practice, 9*(4), 13S–17S.

6. Sturges, D. L. (1994). Communicating through crisis: A strategy for organizational survival. *Management Communication Quarterly, 7*(3), 297–316.

7. Covello, V. T. (2002, October). *Message mapping, risk and crisis communication.* Invited paper presented at the World Health Organization Conference on Bio-terrorism and Risk Communication, Geneva, Switzerland.

8. Covello, V. T. (2003). Best practices in public health risk and crisis communication. *Journal of Health Communication, 8*, 5–8.

9. European Food Safety Authority. (2016). *Best practices for crisis communicators: How to communicate during food or feed safety events.* Parma, Italy: EFSA Publications Office. doi:10.2805/943501

10. Penta, S., Marlowe, V. G., Gill, K., & Kendra, J. (2017). Of earthquakes and epidemics: Examining the applicability of the all-hazards approach in public health emergencies. *Risk, Hazards, & Crisis in Public Policy, 8*(1), 48–67.

11. Peters, R. G., Covello, V. T., & McCallum, D. B. (1997). The determinants of trust and credibility in environmental risk communication: An empirical study. *Risk Analysis, 17*(1), 43–54.

12. Clendenin, A. (2017). The value of source credibility and trust in emergencies and disasters. Unpublished dissertation. Retrieved from oaktrust.library.tamu.edu/handle/1969.1/161542

13. Federal Emergency Management Agency. (2013). Public affairs support annex. Retrieved from https://www.fema.gov/media-library/assets/documents/32276

14. Amadeo, K. (2018). Hurricane Harvey facts, damage and costs. *The Balance.* Retrieved from https://www.thebalance.com/hurricane-harvey-facts-damage-costs-4150087

15. Griggs, B. (September 1, 2017). Harvey's devastating impact by the numbers. *CNN U.S. Edition.* Retrieved from https://www.cnn.com/2017/08/27/us/harvey-impact-by-the-numbers-trnd /index.html

16. Federal Emergency Management Agency. (2017). Historic response to Hurricane Harvey in Texas. Retrieved from https://www.fema.gov/news-release/2017/09/22/historic-disaster -response-hurricane-harvey-texas

17. Hegar, G. (2018). A storm to remember: Hurricane Harvey and the Texas economy. *Fiscal Notes.* Office of the Texas Comptroller of Public Accounts. Retrieved from https://comptroller .texas.gov/economy/fiscal-notes/2018/special-edition/

18. Sebastian, T., Lendering, K., Brand, A. D., Jonkman, S. N., van Gelder, P. H. A. J. M., Godfroij, M., ... Nespeca, V. (2017). *Hurricane Harvey report: A fact-finding effort in the direct aftermath of Hurricane Harvey in the Greater Houston region.* Delft, Netherlands: Delft University Publishers.

19. Rodriguez, R. (2017). Hurricane Harvey contaminates livestock water supplies. *KRIS-TV.* Retrieved from https://animalscience.tamu.edu/2017/09/13/hurricane-harvey -contaminates-livestock-water-supplies/

20. Smith, J., Banik, S., & Haque, U. (2018). Catastrophic hurricanes and public health dangers: Lessons learned. *Journal of Public Health and Emergency, 2*(7). doi: 10.21037/jphe.2018.01.04

21. Horney, J. A., Casillas, G. A., Baker, E., Stone, K. W., Kirsch, K., Camarago, K., ... McDonald, T. J. (2018). Comparing residential contamination in a Houston environmental justice neighborhood before and after Hurricane Harvey. *PLoS One, 13*(2), 1–16.

22. Hellerstedt, J. (2017). Public health and healthcare response to Hurricane Harvey. Presentation to House Committee on Appropriations. Retrieved from https://www.dshs.texas.gov /legislative/2017-Reports/DSHS-HAC10022017.pptx

23. Janssen, M., Lee, J., Bharosa, N., & Cresswell, A. (2010). Advances in multi-agency disaster management: key elements in disaster research. *Information Systems Frontiers, 12*, 1–7.

CHAPTER 19

Get Fit for Health: Using Service Learning to Teach Students How to Address Physical Activity and Healthy Eating Among African American Congregants

Moya L. Alfonso, PhD, MSPH
Abraham Johnson, MPH
Jannapha Hubeny, BSPH
Maria Olivas, MPH

▶ Background

O besity is major health crisis in the United States. According to the National Center for Health Statistics 2017 Brief, between 2015 and 2016, an estimated 39.8% of the U.S. adult population was obese.[1] Among adults 20 years and older, non-Hispanic blacks (46.8%) and Hispanics (47.0%) are disproportionately impacted with obesity compared to non-Hispanic Whites (37.9%).[1] The Healthy People 2020 initiative recommends balancing a healthy diet and engaging in regular physical activity to decrease obesity.[2] In 2014, only about 51% of adults in the state of Georgia engaged in at least 150 minutes of moderate or vigorous physical activity per week.[3] In addition, in Georgia, non-Hispanic Blacks have a higher prevalence of obesity (38.8%) compared to Whites (31.8%), even though the latter are the least physically active.[3] Lack of physical activity and poor eating habits among African Americans have been associated with issues related to self-perception[4] and support.[5]

To increase African Americans' participation in physical activity, studies have evaluated perceptions about obesity, exercising, and social support. In one study, African American women of various weights perceived the word "obesity" as having a negative connotation or as being associated with something abnormal.[4] Also, stress, time, culture, and financial resources were viewed as contributing factors to issues related with their weight.[4] Older African American female church-goers perceived that physical activity required effort, was beneficial to maintaining optimal physical mobility, helped them stay busy, and supported their mental well-being.[6] Similarly, among African American women with type 2 diabetes, social support and self-efficacy were positive correlated with physical activity.[5] In addition, self-perception of obesity and physical exercise affected eating and physical exercise habits,[4,5] whereas safety, access to and availability of resources, feeling tired after exercising, and lack of motivation were noted as environmental barriers to physical activity.[5,6]

Lack of exposure to nutritional education and social support to maintain a healthy weight decreased willingness to seek medical attention for weight-related problems.[7] Conversely, application of culturally relevant interventions to decrease obesity has been suggested as a more effective approach for the African American community.[8] For example, church-based interventions designed to employ nutritional education (e.g., healthy eating, reading labels, obesity) and physical activity have been shown to empower individuals to improve their diets and exercise habits.[9,10]

The focus of this case is on health education interventions designed to address healthy eating and physical activity among African American adults and youth who attend the Truth and Spirit Worship Center in Statesboro, Georgia, and their demonstration of the CEPH MPH Competencies.

▶ Case Study

Service learning using university–community partnerships is a well-known instructional strategy that enhances student learning of course content and results in professional development through the attainment of real-world experiences and skills; it is an excellent method for ensuring students meet CEPH MPH competencies upon graduation.[11-14] In mid-fall semester 2017, Dr. Moya Alfonso met with Pastor Paul Johnson of the Truth and Spirit Worship Center as a part of another research project. During this meeting, Dr. Alfonso became excited about the potential to assist the worship center in providing health education to its congregation after hearing a description of their health-related conditions and needs. According to Pastor Johnson, diabetes, overweight/obesity, heart disease, marijuana use (among youth), and lack of physical activity were common among adult and youth congregation members. It was during this initial meeting that a university–community partnership took root. During the semester, Dr. Alfonso was teaching three courses at the graduate and undergraduate levels. The following sections describe service learning projects in two courses: Community Health Analysis and Modifying Health Behavior.

Adult Health Education Component

Development of the adult health education began in mid-October with an initial interview with Pastor Johnson at his barbershop. During the interview, students focused on two pertinent questions: (1) What is the biggest health need of your congregation? and (2) What are some of the health behaviors that your congregation struggles with? According to Pastor Johnson, the biggest health need of the congregation was weight maintenance, and the congregation struggled with eating healthy, exercising properly, and operating Fitbit watches correctly.

Developing the Get Fit for Health Intervention

Through student introductions at the beginning of semester, it was established that the Community Health Analysis class was composed of students with backgrounds in fitness, nutrition, and health education. For example, one student, Miranda Price, was a certified personal trainer (CPT). Collectively, the class, with the instructor's approval, decided that the intervention would consist of a culturally tailored health education presentation on the following topics:

- Risk factors associated with inactivity and unhealthy eating
- Easy at-home exercises
- Tips on proper usage of fitness applications
- Tips and recommendations on alternatives to soul food and health substitutions
- Video on vegan soul food
- Tips and recommendations on foods to incorporate in the church's New Year's fast

The name of the intervention, "Get Fit for Health," was voted on by the class. Also included in the intervention was a competition called "The Biggest Maintainer." Participants in the competition were members of the congregation who participated in the intervention. After they listened to the presentation, participants' weights were recorded and they were given the option to set their own goal to either lose weight or maintain their weight over the holiday season; this goal was selected based on the stages of change theory.[15] The class recognized how challenging it can be to lose weight during the holiday season, so they gave participants the option to choose. Participants were weighed again after the holiday season, and first-, second-, and third-place prizes were given to participants who met their goals. The first-place winner received a Fitbit, and the second- and third-place winners received hand weights. At the final weigh-in, participation prizes were given to all participants, including a vegan soul food cookbook developed by the class.

Youth Health Education

In the Modifying Health Behavior course, students created social marketing public service announcements (PSA) targeting physical activity and healthy eating among middle school and high school African American children. The PSAs sought to inform youth of the benefits of physical activity and healthy eating, and suggested solutions to barriers that might be associated with health behaviors in these areas. The following section describes the development of a PSA specific to the benefits of physical activity.

Social Marketing PSA Video

The social marketing tool of choice was a video PSA. Data gathered to develop the plan and provide statistical information were derived from the Youth Risk Behavior Survey (2016). The stages of change theory was also applied to enhance the targeted behavior.[15]

The following statistical information was included in the video to educate adolescents on physical activity levels among youth in the United States and South Carolina:

- In South Carolina, 20.6% of youth do not participate in at least 60 minutes of physical activity (PA) on at least one day.
- Nationwide, 14.3% of youth do not participate in at least 60 minutes of PA on at least one day.
- In South Carolina, 80% of youth do participate in at least 60 minutes of PA on at least one day.

The use of the theoretical framework further illuminated which actions to improve. Because the majority of adolescents already participated in at least 60 minutes of psychical activity on at least one day, the objective was to preserve the activity level (action) and maintain (maintenance) the 60 minutes of physical activity on at least one day.

The video began by stating the data listed previously, along with the need to engage in at least 60 minutes of physical activity per day. The video then listed benefits, barriers, and solutions for achieving that objective. The benefits from performing the recommended behavior included looking better, making lifelong friends, increasing self-esteem, having better overall health, decreasing weight gain, preventing cardiovascular diseases and other related illnesses such as diabetes, decreasing stress, and building muscle growth. The costs of and barriers to physical activity consisted of having little time commitment to physical activity, transportation difficulties, financial barriers, and having no resources to work out or implement the physical activity. In turn, strategies offered to the target audience to lower costs and overcome these barriers consisted of working out at home, watching home workout videos, going to the park, playing sports with friends, joining the Young Men's Christian Association (YMCA) or team sports, joining after-school programs, and using technology to find resources and videos to promote physical activity. A humorous tone was used to attract youth attention and engage youth in considering changing their physical activity behaviors. Overall, the social marketing PSA was a crucial tool in advocating and promoting physical activity among the general population.

Summary Points

1. Most adults and youth in the United States are not getting enough physical activity.
2. Culturally tailoring interventions makes them more successful.

3. Interventions should be theoretically based and target risk factors.
4. Faith-based organizations are in need of public health interventions.

▶ Application of CEPH MPH Competencies

This case study addresses CEPH competencies 9, 18, 19, and 20.

Competency 9: Design a Population-Based Policy, Program, Project, or Intervention

Both courses described in this case study were designed to ensure CEPH competency, which is consistent with Bennett and Walston's recommendation to design public health courses with CEPH competencies in mind.[16] Students who designed PSAs were taught how to "identify basic theories, concepts and models from a range of social and behavioral disciplines that are used in public health research and practice." Through the culminating assignment, they were required to apply these theories to the development of PSAs that addressed physical activity and healthy eating among African American youth.

Competency 18: Select Communication Strategies for Different Audiences and Sectors

In this task, students used Youth Risk Behavior Survey data to "identify the causes of social and behavioral factors that affect health of individuals and populations," a key social and behavioral sciences CEPH competency, and used data to select communication strategies for the target audience—African American youth. Through the use of multimedia, students developed PSAs that demonstrated "oral skills for communicating with different audiences in the context of professional public health activities," thereby addressing health disparities among African American youth. In the Community Health and Analysis course, Dr. Alfonso offered students a choice between designing a health intervention for the Worship Center or taking a traditional final exam. Dr. Alfonso believed that meeting the needs of the congregation would serve as a culminating experience for students and would benefit them more than a traditional final exam and reinforce acquisition of CEPH competencies.

Competency 19: Communicate Audience-Appropriate Public Health Content, Both in Writing and Through Oral Presentation

Service learning is a powerful instructional strategy that requires the application of classroom instruction to real-world settings.[11-14] Combining service learning with public health instruction enables students to apply theory-based knowledge to community settings, which increases their knowledge acquisition.[17-20] Student outcomes of service learning include increased self-efficacy and greater course satisfaction.[21]

Further, service learning participation increases students' local health knowledge and understanding of contributing factors to health, public health policy, and cultural determinants of health.[22] In addition, Parks, McClellan, and McGee suggest that public health students who comprehend determinants of health disparities have increased odds of becoming lifelong health advocates.[20]

In this case study, service learning was used as the primary instructional strategy for ensuring student acquisition of CEPH competencies, including demonstration of "effective written and oral skills for communicating with different audiences in the context of professional public health activities." In designing the interventions, students used a variety of media and strategies to educate community members, including youth, on physical activity and health eating. The activities selected were based on cultural aspects of the target groups.

Competency 20: Describe the Importance of Cultural Competence in Communicating Public Health Content

The students became excited about developing a multimodal health intervention that targeted healthy eating and physical activity among adults. Initially, Pastor Johnson had wanted to target adult males only, but the class decided that African American females play a key role in men's health, so the focus was expanded to include females. Dr. Alfonso met all eight students at Pastor Johnson's barbershop for further discussion of the project and cultural aspects of the target audience that would ultimately impact program success (e.g., food preferences, cooking approaches, physical activity preferences). After that meeting, students were encouraged to take the lead on the project, developing a PowerPoint presentation, a healthy soul food cookbook, and designing a Holiday Weight Maintenance contest, which was selected based on the difficulty of losing weight over the holiday season. The following semester, students returned with the instructor's supervision, weighed participants, and distributed prizes. Reactions to the faith-based public health effort were positive, and most participants were successful in reaching their weight-related goals.

Discussion Questions

1. What incentives can be offered to students and community members for their participation in service learning projects?
2. What are the best strategies for teaching students how to design and implement health education and promotion interventions in a way that ensures cultural competence?
3. How could social media have been used in this service learning project to deliver health education to adults and youth and reinforce acquisition of CEPH competencies?

▶ Acknowledgments

The following students also assisted with the projects: Jeanna Fleming, Alexis George, Michel'Le Hull, Christian Johnson, Dallas McClellan, Miranda Price, Kayla Pruitt, Dustyn Sloan, Amanda Smith, Rosemarie Sullivan, and Kayla Woody.

References

1. Centers for Disease Control and Prevention. (2018). Adult obesity facts. Retrieved from https://www.cdc.gov/obesity/data/adult.html

2. Office of Disease Prevention and Health Promotion. (2018). Healthy People 2020: Nutrition, physical activity, and obesity. Retrieved from https://www.healthypeople.gov/2020/leading-health-indicators/2020-lhi-topics/Nutrition-Physical-Activity-and-Obesity

3. Centers for Disease Control and Prevention. (2014). *2014 state indicator report on physical activity*. Atlanta, GA: US Department of Health and Human Services. Retrieved from https://www.cdc.gov/physicalactivity/downloads/pa_state_indicator_report_2014.pdf

4. López, I. A., Boston, P. Q., Dutton, M., Jones, C. G., Mitchell, M. M., & Vilme, H. (2014). Obesity literacy and culture among African American women in Florida. *American Journal of Health Behavior, 38*(4), 541–552.

5. Komar-Samardzija, M., Braun, L. T., Keithley, J. K., & Quinn, L. T. (2012). Factors associated with physical activity levels in African-American women with type 2 diabetes. *Journal of the American Association of Nurse Practitioners, 24*(4), 209–217.

6. Kosma, M., Buchanan, D., & Hondzinski, J. M. (2016). Complexity of exercise behavior among older African American 2omen. *Journal of Aging and Physical Activity,* 1–41.

7. Ma, M., & Ma, A. (2015). Racial/ethnic differences in knowledge of personal and target levels of cardiovascular health indicators. *Journal of Community Health, 40*(5), 1024–1030.

8. Hill, J. L., You, W., & Zoellner, J. M. (2014). Disparities in obesity among rural and urban residents in a health disparate region. *BMC Public Health, 14*(1), 1051.

9. Martinez, D. J., Turner, M. M., Pratt-Chapman, M., Kashima, K., Hargreaves, M. K., Dignan, M. B., & Hébert, J. R. (2016). The effect of changes in health beliefs among African-American and rural White church congregants enrolled in an obesity intervention: A qualitative evaluation. *Journal of Community Health, 41*(3), 518525.

10. Thomson, J. L., Goodman, M. H., & Tussing-Humphreys, L. (2015). Diet quality and physical activity outcome improvements resulting from a church-based diet and supervised physical activity intervention for rural, Southern, African American adults: Delta Body and Soul III. *Health Promotion Practice, 16*(5), 677–688.

11. Bransford, J., Brown, A., & Cocking, A. (Eds.). (1999). *How people learn: Brain, mind, experience, and school* (Report of the National Research Council). Washington, DC: National Academy Press.

12. Furco, A. (2002). Is service-learning really better than community service? A study of high school service program outcomes. In A. Furco & S. H. Billig (Eds.), *Service learning: The essence of the pedagogy* (pp. 23–52). Greenwich, CT: Information Age Publishers.

13. Klute, M. M., & Billig, S. H. (2002). *The impact of service-learning on MEAP: A large-scale study of Michigan learn and serve grantees*. Denver, CO: RMC Research Corporation.

14. Morgan, W., & Streb, M. (2001). Building citizenship: How quality service-learning develops civic values. *Social Science Quarterly, 82*(1), 154–169.

15. Prochaska, J. O., & DiClemente, C. C. (1982). Transtheoretical therapy: Toward a more integrative model of change. *Psychotherapy: Theory, Research & Practice, 19*(3), 276–288.

16. Bennett, C. J., & Walston, S. (2015). Improving the use of competencies in public health education. *American Journal of Public Health, 105*(suppl 1), S65–S67.

17. Ayub, R. A., Jaffery, T., Aziz, F., & Rahmat, M. (2015). Improving health literacy of women about iron deficiency anemia and civic responsibility of students through service learning. *Education for Health, 28*(2), 130.

18. Florence, J., & Behringer, B. (2011). Community as classroom: Teaching and learning public health in rural Appalachia. *Journal of Public Health Management and Practice, 17*(4), 316–323.

19. Lindsey, B. J., & Hawk, C. W. (2013). Training community health students to develop community-requested social marketing campaigns: An innovative partnership. *Progress in Community Health Partnerships, 7*(2), 219–229.

20. Parks, M. H., McClellan, L. H., & McGee, M. L. (2015). Health disparity intervention through minority collegiate service learning. *Journal of Health Care for the Poor and Underserved, 26*(1), 287–292.

21. Hou, S. I. (2009). Service learning + new Master of Public Health student= challenges for the professor. *International Journal of Teaching and Learning in Higher Education, 20*(2), 292–297.

22. Sabo, S., de Zapien, J., Teufel-Shone, N., Rosales, C., Bergsma, L., & Taren, D. (2015). Service learning: A vehicle for building health equity and eliminating health disparities. *American Journal of Public Health, 105*(suppl 1), S38–S43. http://doi.org/10.2105 /AJPH.2014.302364

CHAPTER 20

Cultural Competence in Healthcare Delivery Among Immigrant Populations in the United States: Identifying and Addressing the Challenges

Elizabeth A. Armstrong-Mensah, PhD, MIA

▶ Background

Increasing population diversity has created both opportunities and challenges for health systems to deliver culturally competent care to the populations they serve. Culturally competent health systems improve health outcomes, provide quality care, respond to the health needs and expectations of the populations they serve, and significantly reduce health disparities. In a world where globalization has eroded national boundaries, and where new and evolving patterns of population movement—including skilled and family migration schemes and humanitarian programs—enable people to migrate, populations, especially those in the developed world, have become diverse.[1] The United States is a developed country with a growing immigrant population. It is one of the most sought-after destinations for international immigrants, with approximately 110,000 migrants entering the country on a daily basis.[2] As the population of the United States becomes more diverse, and as immigrant populations bring their cultures to bear on healthcare delivery, cultural competence on the part of health systems and healthcare providers in the United States becomes very important.

Culture and Health

Culture may be defined as those patterns relative to behavior and the product of human action, which may be inherited and passed on from generation to generation independent of biological genes.[3] Culture is a dynamic force that affects all facets of human life. It is central to human health and health-seeking behavior. It affects perceptions of health and illness, determines how people or a group perceive health and illness, and influences the extent to which people will seek treatment or even use health facilities in times of ill health.[4]

Cultural Competence and Healthcare Delivery

From a healthcare perspective, cultural competence goes beyond cultural dissimilarities. It is the ability of health systems to improve upon the health and well-being of populations by integrating culture into the delivery of healthcare services,[5] and by providing individuals with different values, beliefs, and behaviors with health services that are tailored to their social, cultural, and linguistic needs.[6] Cultural competence allows health systems to operate in ways that reduce barriers to patient care, view health issues from the perspective of their patients, and to be respectful, unassuming, open-minded, and flexible in their healthcare approaches, initiatives, and interventions.[7] Cultural competence enables health systems to respond to the health needs of people of all cultures in a way that upholds their worth and dignity. Additionally, it helps to improve health outcomes, increase the efficiency of clinical and support staff, and create greater patient satisfaction with services rendered.[8]

Cultural Competence Challenges in Healthcare Delivery

In the United States, challenges associated with the delivery of healthcare services to immigrant populations occur at two levels: at the immigrant population level and at the healthcare provider level. Challenges at the immigrant population level include religious beliefs; cultural practices; perceptions about preventive health, disease diagnosis, and treatment; language; and diet. At the provider level, challenges include poor doctor–patient communication, a directive style of care, provision of limited health information, minimum immigrant patient engagement in discussions about treatment options, and overt prejudice.[9] The result is often poor quality of care and negative health outcomes for immigrants.[10] Identifying the challenges associated with immigrant population healthcare delivery in the United States, and the willingness of health systems to take action to address those challenges, is a positive step toward remedying the issue.

▶ Case Study

This case study is based on real-life situations. For the sake of confidentiality, the actual names of the healthcare provider and patients have been removed.

Dr. X is an internist at a private clinic in the United States. She provides comprehensive medical care and works with adults who develop simple or complex problems with their internal organs, including the stomach, kidney, liver, and digestive tract. Dr. X sees both U.S.-born and immigrant patients. Her patients present with acute illnesses such as influenza and chronic diseases including diabetes and hypertension. Some of her patients also present with chronic problems with their eyes, ears, and reproductive systems, as well as digestive difficulties. Dr. X has practiced medicine for over 20 years in both public and private health systems. She practices with a colleague.

Patient A, a 32-year-old Hispanic woman, visits Dr. X at her health facility. Patient A is a stay-at-home mother with two children. Dr. X examines her and finds out that she has type 2 diabetes. Dr. X uses the rest of the consultation period to talk to Patient A about her eating habits and what she can do to manage her diabetes. Upon questioning Patient A, Dr. X finds out that she is eating a lot of carbohydrate-based foods on a regular basis (burritos, beans, white rice, tortillas, chips, and tacos). Dr. X tells Patient A that her diet is high in processed carbohydrates and asks her to limit her consumption of those foods. Dr. X recommends whole-grain options including brown rice, maize, oatmeal, and whole-wheat flour, which have less carbohydrates. Patient A is concerned about the adjustments she has to make to her diet. The foods she is being asked to avoid are all she knows; she cannot see herself eating the foods Dr. X is recommending.

After a few weeks, Patient A goes back to see Dr. X for a follow-up visit. Her condition has not improved. Dr. X discovers that Patient A has not been compliant with her medical treatment and diet. When Dr. X asks Patient A why she is not following her prescribed diet, she states that she has to eat what her mother and grandmother prepare at home. Dr. X asks Patient A to bring her mother and grandmother to her next appointment so they can be educated on the needed changes to make to her diet. There is much resistance to the suggested dietary changes when the two elderly women arrive. They insist that Patient A's diabetes is due to "susto" (folk illness) and not diabetes. Dr. X is surprised to hear that.

Patient B is of Hispanic descent. She is a 28-year-old woman who visits Dr. X about a reproductive health issue. Because she has difficulty communicating in English, she visits Dr. X with her child, who is in the seventh grade and speaks English fluently. The child misses school that day. During the visit, Patient B's child attempts to communicate her mother's symptoms and health concerns to Dr. X, and then tries to translate Dr. X's questions and responses to her mother. There are difficulties at certain points—the child is unable to accurately translate the medical terms associated with reproductive health that Dr. X is using—so she tells her mother what she thinks Dr. X is saying. There is a lot of back-and-forth between mother and child. Dr. X senses the child's difficulties and tries to communicate with Patient B, but it is a struggle. Dr. X neither speaks nor understands Spanish.

Patient C is a 28-year-old Mexican female who works at a restaurant. She visits Dr. X's colleague at the health facility. She complains that she has been experiencing a fever, chills, fatigue, and headaches for several days. Dr. X's colleague gives Patient C a prescription for her condition. After a few days, Patient C returns to the health facility. This time, she wants to see Dr. X. She tells Dr. X that her colleague did not treat her properly the last time she was there, so she did not take the medicine he prescribed. Upon further questioning, Patient C explains that when she lived in Mexico, she was usually given an injection when she had a fever. She did not believe that she received the right treatment from Dr. X's colleague. Patient C says she did not know how to express her concern during her visit. Her English is limited. She tells Dr. X that her colleague did not try to engage her in conversation about her treatment options when he attended to her.

Summary Points

1. The case study presents scenarios of immigrant patient and healthcare provider interactions in the United States.
2. It draws attention to the importance of cultural norms and values in healthcare, and to instances of cultural incompetence in healthcare delivery to immigrant populations in the United States.
3. The case study sets the stage for discussions on cultural competence issues in healthcare delivery to immigrant populations in the United States.

▶ Application of CEPH MPH Competencies

This case study addresses CEPH competencies 20 and 18.

Competency 20: Describe the Importance of Cultural Competence in Communicating Public Health Content

Cultural competence in communication is critical to all aspects of healthcare delivery and the ability of immigrant populations in the United States to assimilate information about their health. It involves communicating with awareness and understanding that sociocultural factors influence health beliefs and health seeking behaviors of immigrant populations. Awareness of this dynamic has implications for reducing disparities in healthcare quality at the provider and health system levels.[11]

Low patient socioeconomic status, language barriers or limited English proficiency, and the inability of healthcare providers to communicate in a culturally competent manner with their immigrant patients about their health and treatment options creates health disparities and negatively impacts immigrant populations' adherence to care, utilization of health services, and satisfaction with healthcare delivery in the United States. Dr. X's interactions with her patients highlight some of these issues.

Dr. X's interaction with Patient A shows her lack of understanding of how immigrant populations perceptions of disease and treatment are influenced by their cultural beliefs and practices. The utilization of culturally competent communication techniques helps to build trust, increase the knowledge of immigrant patient epidemiology and treatment, and, in turn, expands healthcare provider's understanding of a patient's behavior and environment. Cultural competence on the part of healthcare providers can lead to the development of tailored preventive care services and public health initiatives for immigrant populations in the United States.[12] To become culturally competent in their communication with their immigrant patients, healthcare providers need to make a conscious effort to be sensitive to issues of diversity. They also need to make it a point to have some general knowledge about the immigrant populations they serve. Unlike Dr. X, they need to integrate their knowledge of each patient's background and beliefs into their professional interactions.

The case study highlights the challenge presented by language and the need for healthcare providers to develop linguistic competency. Knowledge of the language of patients allows healthcare providers and patients to work together and to discuss health concerns. This was not the case in Dr. X's interaction with Patient B: Language was a problem. Dr. X's inability to speak her patient's language limited Patient B's ability to meaningfully discuss her health concerns and issues. Healthcare providers have their own culture and language, which often affects their interactions with patients.[13] Their inability to effectively communicate health information compels immigrant populations to deal with health situations that are confusing, frustrating, and stressful on their own. This was the situation with Patient B in the case study. A linguistically competent healthcare provider understands the intrinsic cultural meaning of a message and is able to elicit and transmit the right cultural response. Linguistic competency of healthcare providers in the United States can contribute to the health literacy of immigrant populations, thereby improving their health outcomes.

Cultural differences can cause miscommunication and misunderstanding in healthcare delivery, which can result in misdiagnoses, missed opportunities for optimal illness management, and dissatisfaction with treatment. Had the first doctor seen by Patient C in Dr. X's practice recognized this fact, Patient C would not have had to visit Dr. X with the same conditions she presented with to her colleague. Healthcare providers' understanding and recognition of the cultural context of an immigrant patient's illness is essential to a successful therapeutic relationship.[13]

Competency 18: Select Communication Strategies for Different Audiences and Communicate Audience-Appropriate Public Health Content, Both in Writing and Through Oral Presentation

Communication is a key ingredient in effective medical care and disease prevention. The communication that takes place during medical visits includes the expressed content of doctors' diagnoses and patients' questions, as well as patients' unexpressed fears, physicians' unspoken but viscerally communicated assumptions, and the dynamic flow of nonverbal expressions— frowns, grimaces, smiles, and head nods.[14] According to Roter and Hall, communication is the fundamental instrument by which the doctor–patient relationship is crafted and by which therapeutic goals are achieved.[14] Patients bring their own beliefs to the medical visit. In their treatment of patients, doctors often assume that they are treating each patient objectively, viewing their ailments or conditions through what they believe to be the impartial lenses of the medical model. However, despite their intentions, theory and research suggest that these assumptions are sometimes inaccurate.[15]

Meaningful communication between physician and patient usually depends on a patient's need to tell a physician about their illness and the physician's desire to listen, diagnose the health issue, and prescribe appropriate treatment options.[16] According to Ashton et al., patients and doctors have different intellects and values[16]; thus, to have a shared understanding of a health situation, they must both obtain and provide each other with information and try to reconcile differences in perspective. This challenge becomes even more important and difficult if the patient and the doctor come from different cultures.[16]

Discussion Questions

1. Why does cultural competence matter in healthcare delivery?
2. What is the role of culturally competent communication in immigrant population healthcare and disease prevention?
3. Which cultural competence challenges did the patient and the healthcare provider have in each of the case study scenarios?
4. What are some of the cultural competencies that Dr. X and her colleague need to be able to deliver effective healthcare services to their immigrant patients? Explain your response.

References

1. Waters, E., Gibbs, L., Rigg, E., Priest, N., Renzaho, A., & Kulkens, M. (2008). Cultural competence in public health. In S. Quah & K. Heggenhougen (Eds.), *International encyclopedia of public health* (pp. 38–44). San Diego, CA: Elsevier/Academic Press.
2. Martin, P. (2013). The global challenge of managing migration. *Population Bulletin, 68*(2), 1–20.
3. Parson, T. (1949). *Essays in sociological theory.* Glencoe, IL: Free Press.
4. Armstrong-Mensah, E. (2017). *Lecture notes: Global health issues, challenges, and global action.* Hoboken, NJ: Wiley-Blackwell.
5. National Health and Medical Research Council. (2006). *Cultural competence in health: A guide for policy, partnerships and participation.* Canberra, Australia: Author.
6. Betancourt, J. R., Green, A. R., & Carrillo, J. E. (2002). *Cultural competence in health care: Emerging frameworks and practical approaches.* New York, NY: Commonwealth Fund.
7. George Town Health Policy Institute. (2004). Cultural competence in health care: Is it important for people with chronic conditions? *Issue Brief 5.* Retrieved from https://hpi .georgetown.edu/agingsociety/pubhtml/cultural/cultural.html
8. Brach, C., & Fraserirector, I. (2000). Can cultural competency reduce racial and ethnic disparities? A review and conceptual model. *Medical Care Research and Review, 57*(1), 181–217.
9. Tello, M. (2017). Racism and discrimination in health care: Providers and patients. Retrieved from https://www.health.harvard.edu/blog/racism-discrimination-health-care-providers -patients-2017011611015
10. Brach, C., Fraser, I., & Paez, K. (2005). Crossing the language chasm: An in-depth analysis of what language-assistance programs look like in practice. *Health Affairs, 24*(2), 424–434. Retrieved from https://www.healthaffairs.org/doi/full/10.1377/hlthaff.24.2.424
11. Taylor, S., & Lurie, N. (2004). The role of culturally competent communication in reducing ethnic and racial healthcare disparities. *American Journal of Managed Care, 10,* SP1–SP4.
12. Brach, C., & Fraser. (2002). Reducing disparities through culturally competent health care: An analysis of the business case. *Quality Management in Health Care, 10*(4), 15–28. Retrieved from https://www.ncbi.nlm.nih.gov/pmc/articles/PMC5094358/pdf/nihms-825244.pdf
13. Health Resources and Services Administration. (2005). Transforming the face of health professions through cultural and linguistic competence education: The role of the HRSA centers of excellence. Retrieved from https://www.hrsa.gov/sites/default/files/culturalcompetence /cultcompedu.pdf
14. Roter, D. L., & Hall, J. (1993). *Doctors talking with patients/patients talking with doctors: Improving communication in medical visits.* Westport, CT: Auburn House.
15. Van Ryn, M., & Burke, J. (2000). The effect of patient race and socio-economic status on physicians' perceptions of patients. *Social Science & Medicine, 50*(6), 813–828.
16. Ashton, C., Haidet, P., Paterniti, D., Collins, T., Gordon, H., & O'Malley, K. (2003). Racial and ethnic disparities in the use of health services: Bias, preferences, or poor communication? *General Internal Medicine, 18,* 146–152.

SECTION 7

Interprofessional Practice and Systems Thinking

CHAPTER 21

Oral Rapid HIV Testing in University-Based Dental Clinics in Metro New York City

Anthony J. Santella, DrPH, MCHES
Gwen Cohen Brown, DDS, FAAOMP

▶ Background

Human immunodeficiency virus (HIV) and other sexually transmitted infections continue to be of public health significance in the United States. At the end of 2015, there were approximately 1.1 million people older than the age of 13 in the United States who were living with HIV. This group includes an estimated 162,000 people (15%) who are living with HIV, but unaware of their status. Despite advances in prevention methods and technologies, we continue to see a static number of new HIV diagnoses. In 2016, 39,782 people were newly diagnosed with HIV.[1]

There are many benefits of knowing your HIV status. First, testing provides an opportunity to be linked to HIV care and treatment, if needed. Individuals living with HIV who are diagnosed soon after infection can live long healthy lives if they are aware of their status and are adherent to their medications.[2] Second, being aware of their HIV status allows individuals to not transmit the virus to their sex partners.[2] We now know that people living with HIV who are adherent to their HIV medication and maintain an undetectable viral load have virtually no chance of sexually transmitting HIV to their partners (a concept known as "undetectable equals untransmittable" or "U=U").[3] Finally, being aware of their HIV status can allow individuals to make informed choices about which prevention tools and technologies best meet their needs (e.g., condoms, pre-exposure prophylaxis [PrEP]).[2]

171

Although the majority of HIV testing takes place in medical facilities, there is a movement to routinize it by bringing it to nontraditional venues such as the dental setting. Oral rapid HIV testing is completed using a relatively simple process. With a third-generation oral HIV test, the provider swabs the patient's buccal mucosa and gingiva. Next, the provider places the end of the swab device in a vial that holds an enzyme solution that reacts to any antibody–antigen binding. As the oral fluid and the enzymes make their way up the test strip, they encounter the HIV–antigen substance. If the oral fluid contains HIV antibodies, they start to bind to the antigens, and the enzyme reacts, causing a color change on the strip. This produces a line on the read-out portion of the device. This line indicates a reaction but is not considered to be a definite positive result. Like all other HIV tests, oral rapid HIV tests require a confirmatory blood test before a patient is considered to be HIV positive.[4]

The dental setting is an untapped venue for conducting oral rapid HIV testing. Dentists and hygienists are already conducting oral exams and routinely conduct screening tests such as those for oral cancer and hypertension. Moreover, we know that a large proportion of Americans regularly attend dental appointments, yet do not receive regular exams from primary care providers.[5] A growing body of literature indicates that both dentists[6-8] and dental hygienists[9,10] are knowledgeable about HIV and willing to conduct the test in the dental clinic environment. Moreover, strong evidence supports that dental patients are also willing to receive oral rapid HIV testing.[11-13]

This case study focuses on an interprofessional research study in which oral rapid HIV testing was implemented in three metro New York City dental clinics staffed by dental hygiene faculty and senior dental hygiene students.

▶ Case Study

The study took place in three public university–based dental clinics in metropolitan New York City. Two of the three dental hygiene clinics are designated as Hispanic-serving institutions, reflecting the local population, while the third is located in a suburban environment. Each site included a dentist, multiple registered dental hygienists, and dental hygiene students. The dentist served as the laboratory director—a position needed to secure a waiver from the State Health Department to conduct screening tests in a setting without a laboratory. The overall project principal investigator (PI) was a public health scientist who works in an academic setting (not part of the three study sites). The final study team member was a statistician/epidemiologist who also works in an academic setting.

The interprofessional team of dentists, dental hygienists, dental hygiene students, HIV clinicians, and public health scientists and educators took approximately a year to plan the study. This planning included development of the study protocol, design of data collection forms, securing of supplies (oral rapid HIV test kits), and going through the institutional review board process at two different university systems. The final part of the planning process was to train those who would be conducting the testing (dental hygienists and senior dental hygiene students) and supervising the testing staff (dentists) who were trained in the basics of HIV prevention, epidemiology/surveillance, and the testing process. Training took place through several media. All study staff reviewed an online module from the test kit manufacturer that explained how the test should be conducted and how the results should be interpreted. The PI also conducted an HIV 101 training with staff to ensure they all were familiar with the basics of HIV (modes of transmission, local epidemiology data, advances in care, treatment, and prevention). The local health department also provided a 1-day training that included practice in offering the test, conducting it, and giving both nonreactive/negative and reactive/positive results.

The program proceeded as follows at all three testing sites. First, recruitment flyers were placed in the dental clinic reception area on designated HIV testing days, which ranged from 1 to 3 days per week, to inform both new and returning patients about the study. Interested patients older than the age of 17 were instructed to approach their dental provider (a senior hygiene student or hygiene faculty member) about receiving the oral rapid HIV test. The study staff provided patients who expressed interest with a consent form; after they signed it, the staff escorted the patients to a remote cubicle location and/or private office setting and took an oral swab with a test kit. Twenty minutes later, the study staff read the result as reactive, nonreactive, or indeterminate; another trained student or faculty study team member provided a second reading before results were shared with the patient. Participants completed a brief questionnaire that captured their demographic characteristics, healthcare utilization, and risk behaviors.

All participants in this study ($n = 231$) received nonreactive test results. Had any been reactive, the hygiene faculty member would have taken a dried blood spot specimen by fingerstick to be sent to the State Public Health Laboratory for Western blot processing (i.e., confirmatory test; as noted earlier, the rapid test is only a screening test and does not confirm an HIV diagnosis). An appointment would have been made within 48 hours of receiving the preliminary reactive result with an HIV-specialist physician at a local designated AIDS center (where each site has an executed memorandum of understanding with the institutions involved in the study) and the patient would have received the results of the confirmatory Western blot test as well as follow-up care, if needed. The hygiene faculty member would have documented the appointment information and the provision of the Western blot test in the patient dental record as per State Department of Health protocol. The designated AIDS center would have had the responsibility of providing the actual HIV diagnosis and providing HIV care and treatment services.

Once the study data collection was complete, all study staff were interviewed by the PI about their experience offering and implementing the oral rapid HIV testing in the dental setting. The interviews, with participant permission, were audio-recorded. Interviews were professionally transcribed and analyzed using a grounded theory approach.

Basic descriptive statistics on the study participants data obtained from the self-administered questionnaires were conducted by the statistician/epidemiologist using Microsoft Excel and SAS. With these data, scientific conference presentations and posters were submitted and prepared to both dental and public health venues. The PI and other study staff conducted qualitative analysis of the study staff interviews, which included line-by-line coding of the interview transcripts. These data were also submitted for publication to both scientific conferences and for peer-reviewed journals.

Summary Points

1. An interprofessional approach is needed to successfully implement a public health intervention using biomedical technology.
2. Clinicians such as dentists and dental hygienists need a deep understanding of public health epidemiology, surveillance, and policies to address clinical issues in a comprehensive fashion.
3. Dentists and dental hygienists are becoming more comfortable with the idea of providing HIV testing, but there is still some resistance in private offices where providers may feel that HIV testing is outside their scope of practice or there may be difficulty in connecting patients to further care.

▶ Application of CEPH MPH Competencies

This case study addresses CEPH competency 21.

Competency 21: Perform Effectively on Interprofessional Teams

Ideally, productive interprofessional collaborations between healthcare providers will increase the efficacy of how health care is both presented to and accepted by the public.[14] Conversely, poor interprofessional collaborations can negatively impact the provision of health care.[15] To be truly interprofessional, health care must to be implemented through a collaborative lens, and providers must work with one another constructively, communicate well, balance all roles in patient care, learn how to resolve differences in approaches to treatment, and minimize power differentials.[15]

Oral healthcare providers are taught to incorporate the presentation of systemic disease into the oral health evaluation of their patients; they recognize that incomplete or inappropriate oral health assessment and screening may lead to detrimental general health consequences, and that systemic disease may develop across an individual's life span. Interprofessional collaborations can be challenging, however, as we are taught to excel within individual fields, in our own academic silos, and are rarely exposed to other disciplines during the course of our studies.

Of concern is the lack of didactic materials taught in medical education regarding the oral–systemic disease connection[16] and how, by using a collaborative approach among dental, medical, and public health professionals, both oral and systemic disease can be diagnosed earlier and treated more effectively.[17] Data amassed from an international study on the inclusion of oral/systemic health in curricula in medical, nursing, and pharmacy programs demonstrate that historically there has been a lack of dental knowledge about this linkage, with only 53.7% of the respondents to the study survey indicating that incorporating this material into current curricula was somewhat important.[16] Notably, none of the schools in the study ranked knowledge of the oral manifestations of HIV as very important.[16] Unless education of medical and dental providers becomes more collaborative at its core, resistance to interprofessional patient care will likely persist.

In addition to educational barriers to interprofessional collaboration, physical and organizational obstacles to such practice exist.[14] Dentists often practice as solo providers, few work in medical centers, and a hospital residency is not required for dental licensure in all states. Dental hygienists have even less interaction with medical providers, as direct contact regarding patient care may be considered outside of their scope of practice. Physicians are often members of a medical team and routinely collaborate interprofessionally with nurses, physician assistants, and other hospital-based clinicians.[15] Conversely, for many years physicians and dentists have operated in two separate worlds, with respect to both education and physical space.[18]

In the *Healthy People 2020* initiative, the current goals under the category of oral health include the "prevention and control of oral and craniofacial diseases, conditions, and injuries, and improve access to preventive services and dental care."[19] The first of the current objectives is to "Increase awareness of the importance of oral health to overall health and well-being."[19] The creation of interprofessional collaborations between public health dentists and medical providers, beginning with the recognition that oral health is essential to overall health, is one way to achieve this goal. Development of methods to increase interactions among healthcare professionals in the clinical setting as well as the educational setting is needed,[19] and is a prerequisite to accomplish the educational objectives included in *Healthy People 2020* using the Education for Health framework.[20]

How can we move forward with public health–oriented projects that focus on collaborative interprofessional clinical care? One example of a successful interprofessional project is HIV testing in a dental care setting. It has been documented that patients are accepting of dentists and dental hygienists initiating and offering HIV testing[7,9] in clinics and private practice, providing that a plan is in place for dealing with a preliminary positive result and the dental providers collaborate with medical providers at a designated AIDS center.[12]

In addition to HIV testing in a dental care setting, successful public health campaigns include those targeting fluoridation and caries reduction, early oral health intervention and Head Start programs, and the oral health concerns of patients with special needs/disabilities.[21] What is known through evaluation of these public health collaborations is that the most effective projects are built around the issues of importance to a specific community and for which all of the participants have a shared stake in the outcome.[21] Partnering with public health professionals can build capacity and facilitate successful outcomes related to specific clinical goals by including expertise in policy development, epidemiology, and program planning.

It is essential that healthcare providers begin to work collaboratively, become familiar with multidisciplinary knowledge, and incorporate research into practice to help propel forward their disciplines and provide thoughtful integrated patient care. Public health professionals can help bridge the educational gaps between providers and facilitate collaborations between differing clinical fields.

When two previously separate concepts are merged into a singular idea, novel properties can emerge that were not present in either of the original components.[22] Public health professionals focusing on interprofessional collaborations can be the forces that unite healthcare providers by creating new solutions to address existing problems. For public health dentistry, interprofessional collaborative care is the future of comprehensive care.

Discussion Questions

1. How can interprofessional collaborative practice be introduced effectively in medical, dental, and allied health programs so that such care is integrated before clinicians graduate?
2. How can public health professionals determine the significant issues affecting specific healthcare communities to create interprofessional campaigns?
3. How can public health professionals reach clinicians outside of academic institutions to assess the changing needs of their professions?

▶ Acknowledgments

We would like to thank the study site coordinators, Susan Davide, MS, MSEd, RDH (NYC College of Technology), Hanna Horowitz, DDS (Farmingdale State College), and Petal Leuwaisee, MS, RDH (Hostos Community College), for their leadership in planning and implementing this study.

References

1. Centers for Disease Control and Prevention. (2018, June 26). HIV/AIDS: Statistics overview. Retrieved from https://www.cdc.gov/hiv/statistics/overview/index.html
2. Centers for Disease Control and Prevention. (2016, August). HIV testing in the United States. Retrieved from https://www.cdc.gov/nchhstp/newsroom/docs/factsheets/hiv-testing-us-508.pdf
3. Prevention Access Campaign. (n.d.). U=U. Retrieved from https://www.preventionaccess.org/
4. OraSure Technologies. (2012, August 1). Infectious disease. Retrieved from http://www.orasure.com/products-infectious/products-infectious.asp
5. Pollack, H. A., Metsch, L. R., & Abel, S. (2010). Dental examinations as an untapped opportunity to provide HIV testing for high-risk individuals. *American Journal of Public Health, 100*(1), 88–89. doi:10.2105/ajph.2008.157230
6. Pollack, H. A., Pereyra, M., Parish, C. L., Abel, S., Messinger, S., Singer, R., . . . Metsch, L. R. (2014). Dentists' willingness to provide expanded HIV screening in oral health care settings: Results from a nationally representative survey. *American Journal of Public Health, 104*(5), 872–880. doi:10.2105/ajph.2013.301700
7. Parish, C. L., Siegel, K., Liguori, T., Abel, S. N., Pollack, H. A., Pereyra, M. R., & Metsch, L. R. (2018). HIV testing in the dental setting: Perspectives and practices of experienced dental professionals. *AIDS Care, 30*(3), 347–352. doi:10.1080/09540121.2017.1367087
8. Shimpi, N., Schroeder, D., Kilsdonk, J., Chyou, P., Glurich, I., & Acharya, A. (2016). Assessment of dental providers' knowledge, behavior and attitude towards incorporating chairside screening for medical conditions: A pilot study. *Journal of Dentistry and Oral Care Medicine, 2*(1), 1–7. doi:10.15744/2454-3276.2.102
9. Santella, A. J., Davide, S. H., Cortell, M., & Tuthill, J. (2012). The role of dental hygienists in conducting rapid HIV testing. *Journal of Dental Hygiene, 86*(4), 265–271.
10. Santella, A. J., Krishnamachari, B., Davide, S. H., Cortell, M., Furnari, W., Watts, B., & Haden, S. (2013). Dental hygienists' knowledge of HIV, attitudes towards people with HIV and willingness to conduct rapid HIV testing. *International Journal of Dental Hygiene, 11*(4), 287–292. doi:10.1111/idh.12022
11. VanDevanter, N., Combellick, J., Hutchinson, M. K., Phelan, J., Malamud, D., & Shelley, D. (2012). A qualitative study of patients' attitudes toward HIV testing in the dental setting. *Nursing Research and Practice, 2012*, 1–6. doi:10.1155/2012/803169

12. Davide, S. H., Santella, A. J., Furnari, W., & Krishnamachari, B. (2017). Patients' willingness to participate in rapid HIV testing: A pilot study in three New York city dental hygiene clinics. *Journal of Dental Hygiene, 91*(6), 41–48.

13. Dietz, C. A., Ablah, E., Reznik, D., & Robbins, D. K. (2008). Patients' attitudes about rapid oral HIV screening in an urban, free dental clinic. *AIDS Patient Care and STDs, 22*(3), 205–212. doi:10.1089/apc.2007.0235

14. D'Amour, D., Ferrada-Videla, M., San Martin Rodriguez, L., & Beaulieu, M. (2005). The conceptual basis for interprofessional collaboration: Core concepts and theoretical frameworks. *Journal of Interprofessional Care, 19*(suppl 1), 116–131. doi:10.1080/13561820500082529

15. Zwarenstein, M., Goldman, J., & Reeves, S. (2009). Interprofessional collaboration: Effects of practice-based interventions on professional practice and healthcare outcomes. *Cochrane Database of Systematic Reviews.* doi:10.1002/14651858.cd000072.pub2

16. Hein, C., Schönwetter, D. J., & Iacopino, A. M. (2011). Inclusion of oral–systemic health in predoctoral/undergraduate curricula of pharmacy, nursing, and medical schools around the world: A preliminary study. *Journal of Dental Education, 75*(9), 1187–1199.

17. Slavkin, H. C., & Bruce, J. B. (2000). Relationship of dental and oral pathology to systemic illness. *Journal of the American Medical Association, 284*(10), 1215–1217. doi:10.1001/jama.284.10.1215

18. Wilder, R. S., O'Donnell, J. A., Barry, J. M., Galli, D. M., Hakim, F. F., Holyfield, J., & Robbins, M. R. (2008). Is dentistry at risk? A case for interprofessional education. *Journal of Dental Education, 72*(11), 1231–1237.

19. Healthy People 2020. (2018, July). Oral health. Retrieved from https://www.healthypeople.gov/2020/topics-objectives/topic/oral-health

20. Zenzano, T., Allan, J. D., Bigley, M. B., Bushardt, R. L., Garr, D. R., Johnson, K., . . . Stanley, J. M. (2011). The roles of healthcare professionals in implementing clinical prevention and population health. *American Journal of Preventive Medicine, 40*(2), 261–267. doi:10.1016/j.amepre.2010.10.023

21. Mouradian, W. E., Huebner, C., & DePaola, D. (2004). Addressing health disparities through dental–medical collaborations, Part III: Leadership for the public good. *Journal of Dental Education, 68*(5), 505–512.

22. Ward, T. B. (2004). Cognition, creativity, and entrepreneurship. *Journal of Business Venturing, 19*(2), 173–188.

CHAPTER 22

A Coordinated, Multisectoral Response to the Opioid Crisis in a High-Overdose Region

Kimberly Krytus, MSW, MPH, CPH

Gale Burstein, MD, MPH, FAAP

▶ Background

With a population of nearly 1 million,[1] Erie County is located in western New York on the banks of Lake Erie; its heart is the state's second largest city, Buffalo. In September 2015, the medical examiner for the Erie County Department of Health (ECDOH) noticed a steep increase in opioid-related deaths, which grew by 27% from 2013 to 2014 and by 100% from 2014 to 2015. Opioid-related deaths peaked in 2016 with 301 deaths, a 30% increase from 2015. This followed a similar trend of increasing opioid-related overdoses and deaths across the United States that began in 2012, becoming a national crisis.[2,3] In Erie County, epidemiologists identified fentanyl as the fastest-growing cause of opioid-related deaths, associated with 76% of fatal overdoses in 2016, up from 27% in 2014. At the same time, law enforcement agencies were increasingly finding fentanyl and heroin throughout cities, towns, and villages. The epidemic affected urban, rural, and suburban neighborhoods alike, and persons of all races, genders, and age groups.[4,5] If it could not be halted, thousands more could lose their lives.

The ECDOH identified many factors contributing to the epidemic. Built on steel and manufacturing industries, Buffalo has a large working-class population.[6] In 2015, the county experienced higher rates of disability and inpatient and outpatient surgeries, and had one of the highest rates of painkiller prescriptions in

New York State.[7] Healthcare leaders recognized that addiction often began with prescription painkillers that progressed to street drugs.

In 2013, the NYS Prescription Monitoring Program (PMP) went into effect. It required most New York State prescribers to consult the Internet System for Tracking Over-Prescribing (I-STOP) PMP registry when prescribing Schedule II, III, and IV controlled substances.[8] The new law reduced opioid prescriptions in general, but especially for persons who were frequenting multiple healthcare providers in a short period of time to fill numerous prescriptions. Those who were no longer able to access prescription opioids from healthcare providers began seeking drugs through other means, including street supplies. At the same time, the heroin supply increased considerably while this drug's cost dramatically decreased, and overdose-related emergency department (ED) visits and opioid-related deaths continued to rise.[9,10]

▶ Case Study

A Multisectoral Task Force Responds

Understanding that no single strategy could effectively halt the epidemic, officials recognized that there was a critical need to coordinate opioid prevention initiatives. In February 2016, County Executive Mark Poloncarz signed Executive Order #014 establishing an Opioid Epidemic Task Force. Co-led by county commissioners of the departments of health and mental health, the task force included experts from social services, law enforcement, provider networks, mental health and addictions, insurers, first responders, educators, community-based organizations, family members, and close friends. The task force established a cross-functional, collaborative framework to guide initiatives (**FIGURE 22-1**) with a mission to develop and share best practices, provide support to individuals and families battling addiction, and deliver community-based prevention and treatment programs.[10,11]

The task force established seven committees to carry out this work. Priorities included changing pain management prescribing practices; expanding rapid access to community-based medication-assisted treatment (MAT); educating, training, and distributing lifesaving naloxone (Narcan®); and eliminating the stigma associated with opioid addiction. Committees met monthly and the entire task force met quarterly to discuss priority areas, and updates were shared with the public.[10]

The *Provider Education and Policy Reform* committee, co-led by an addictions medicine physician and the county health commissioner, developed local acute pain

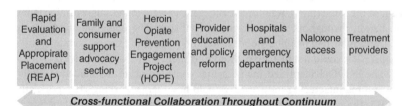

FIGURE 22-1 Opiate overdose continuum cross-functional collaboration in Erie County.

Reproduced from: Erie County Department of Health. (2018). Opiate epidemic task force. Retrieved from http://www2.erie.gov/health/index.php?q=opiate-epidemic -task-force

management guidelines, trained more than 200 providers to prescribe buprenor-phine, and established new methadone sites and adolescent MAT clinics, quickly expanding MAT access.[10] They also collaborated with the Erie County Medical Society and the New York State American Academy of Pediatrics to roll out Screening, Brief Intervention and Referral to Treatment (SBIRT), a comprehensive and integrated intervention and treatment program for providers to identify and treat addiction early,[12] and worked with health plans to reimburse SBIRT.[10] To counter myths and address stigma, they created two public service announcements that aired in movie theaters and on websites.[10]

The *Community Education and Prevention* committee, led by a representative of the U.S. Attorney General's Office, generated community awareness of the opioid epidemic and created prevention programs, launching them with a number of key audiences including schools and courts. Committee members surveyed schools to understand their anti-opioid educational activities, and developed and shared an opioid prevention curriculum with school superintendents across western New York. To increase awareness, they obtained funding to launch a large billboard campaign with anti-stigma and MAT endorsement messages.

Led by a parent advocate who lost her son to addiction, the *Families and Consumer Support and Advocacy* committee brought attention to the epidemic by hosting events such as Personal Experience Speaker Groups, Overdose Awareness Days, grief support groups, and memorials. They also launched awareness campaigns for an opioid abuse hotline, and lobbied for more treatment facilities and harsher sentences for predatory drug dealers.[10]

Collaborating with law enforcement, the *Rapid Evaluation for Appropriate Placement (REAP)* program connected those who voluntarily came to a police station to treatment services. The county sheriff's department and police departments for the city of Buffalo and its largest surrounding suburbs, covering more than 70% of the county's population, participated in REAP.[10] In 2017, the ECDOH and the Cheektowaga Police, one of the largest local police units in the region, worked with peer educators to pilot an initiative advising overdose survivors on harm-reduction and MAT services. Using ODMAP, a database that tracks overdoses and first responder naloxone use in real time, police and peer educators contacted overdose survivors 2 to 3 days following their overdose resuscitation and discussed harm-reduction and MAT options. Following a successful pilot, the program expanded in 2018, linking other local police departments to peer counselors to advise overdose victims on MAT and harm reduction in western New York.[10]

The *Substance Abuse Treatment Providers* committee, led by the county commissioner of mental health and the director of a large behavioral health and substance use treatment network, expanded treatment access by launching an addictions hotline that provided referrals and support to individuals and their families and linked them to outpatient care, peer services, and family support. By 2017, MAT community demand and access had increased dramatically. Local treatment providers enhanced MAT effectiveness, offering rapid access by starting medications within 24 to 48 hours of the first appointment. With New York State funding, one of the largest local providers developed 24/7 open access centers delivering immediate engagement, assessment, and referral services for people suffering from addiction. Helping to plan this initiative, the committee facilitated collaborations across systems that included medical care, hospitals, peer and family advocate organizations, and state and local governments.[10]

Recognizing that the court system was incarcerating individuals for substance use, the city of Buffalo established the nation's first opioid crisis court in May 2017 to fast-track defendants into treatment,[13] linking them with providers who could offer MAT, including methadone or buprenorphine the same or next day. The committee also worked with local judges to combat the criminal stigma of addiction; promoted compassion and evidence-based addictions management, including MAT; and drafted a statement on stigma that was shared with multiple audiences across the community.[10]

The *Hospitals/ED* committee, led by an ED physician, collaborated with 14 hospitals to administer naloxone, dispense naloxone for home use to overdose cases seen in the ED, launch an ED buprenorphine induction and rapid treatment referral pilot, and educate hospitalists to continue admitted patients on MAT in the hospital. To aid in care coordination, they built treatment referrals into the local EDs' electronic medical record (EMR) systems.[10,14]

Led by an ECDOH medical care administrator, the *Naloxone Access* committee focused on community education, training, and distribution of lifesaving medication. Between 2014 and 2018, more than 700 community-based naloxone trainings were held at fire departments, community and senior centers, libraries, colleges, and churches. By June 2018, more than 6000 community members and more than 15,000 first responders had been trained in administering naloxone. The committee also increased the number of drug disposal kiosks in EDs and in the community.[10]

The task force was highly collaborative in its efforts, leveraging expertise from all sectors and constituent groups. In 2017, opioid-related deaths decreased for the first time since 2013, dropping to 251, down from 301 deaths in 2016. As of November 2018, deaths for that year were trending to drop below 200, a further decline of 20%.[10] While acknowledging that the number of deaths remains unacceptably high, County Executive Poloncarz stated that "this is a tremendous sign that the work we have been doing in our community over the last two years is making a difference." Further, hydrocodone prescribed for Medicaid recipients, previously the number one prescribed drug in the county, dropped to number ten, demonstrating success on multiple fronts. "This is an all-hands-on-deck fight, but we are seeing progress,"[5] said Poloncarz, adding that "despite progress there is no time to rest; as long as opioid addiction and overdose continue to take lives in western New York, the work of the task force continues" (personal communication, June 19, 2018).

Summary Points

1. ECDOH recognized the significant increases in opioid deaths in 2015, and subsequently created a multisectoral Opiate Epidemic Task Force to address the crisis.

2. The task force collaborated with families, first responders, communities, providers, insurers, local organizations, law enforcement, and courts to prioritize evidence-based prevention, treatment, education, and policy interventions addressing key contributing factors.

3. County leaders brought stakeholders together, created a vision and collaborative framework, and empowered the task force to combat factors that increased mortality.

4. Opioid-related deaths dropped in 2017 for the first time in 5 years, reversing the trend.

▶ Application of CEPH MPH Competencies

This case study addresses CEPH competencies 22 and 13.

Competency 22: Apply Systems Thinking Tools to a Public Health Issue

The task force viewed the opioid crisis as a system of interrelationships between policy-makers, providers, individuals, communities, first responders, law enforcement, and courts, which were all connected in ways that fueled the epidemic. By applying systems thinking tools, the members gained understanding of the causes and effects of the various factors, and changes occurring in the system over time.[15]

When deaths spiked in 2015, county leaders recognized that the structure of the opioid-related system generated a pattern of responses from providers, individuals, law enforcement, and others that unintentionally increased opioid use, overdose, and death. By applying stocks, flows, and feedback loops (tools for systems thinking), they could identify points to intervene and alter the system's trajectory. **FIGURE 22-2** presents the opioid system's *stocks,* or variables that accumulated over time (boxes); *flows,* or links between variables (wide arrows); factors that flowed into or increased stocks (circles); and intervention pathways (dotted lines).

Feedback loops revealed the factors influencing the system (Figure 22-2). Reinforcing factors (narrow solid lines) applied positive feedback to the system, increasing deaths. For example, while I-STOP reduced prescriptions, it contributed to increased illicit drug use, which then increased overdose and death rates. As a single system change, I-STOP did not alter the system's trajectory. By viewing the whole system, however, the task force could see multiple points to intervene. Police and courts prioritized treatment. Providers adopted MAT and SBIRT and expanded access to buprenorphine and methadone therapies. Community-based organizations, advocates, and support networks focused on awareness and education, launched a hotline, and addressed myths and stigma, and the county scaled up naloxone training of first responders and community members. These interventions

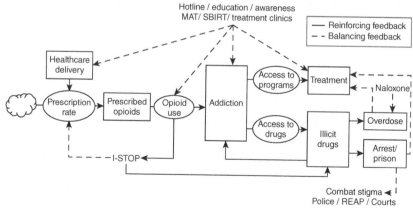

FIGURE 22-2 Stock and flow map and feedback loops of the opioid system.

(dotted lines) applied negative feedback to balance the system, altering its trajectory and reducing deaths.

Competency 13: Propose Strategies to Identify Stakeholders and Build Coalitions and Partnerships for Influencing Public Health Outcomes

The ECDOH coalition influenced policy-makers, police, courts, providers, and communities to expand and rapidly deploy MAT and SBIRT, link individuals to treatment services early, combat the stigma of addiction, train responders and distribute naloxone, and establish and promote the addiction hotline throughout the region.

The task force also applied principles of leadership, governance, and management by creating a vision, empowering others, fostering collaboration, and guiding decision making. Its members focused their efforts on reducing mortality, creating a vision of a community in which no one died as a result of an opioid overdose, and a framework that promoted collaborative decision making and empowered committees to act toward their vision.[10,15,16] Effective collaboration and leadership helped balance the system, ultimately contributing to reductions in the number of opioid-related deaths.

Discussion Questions

1. Which task force interventions were key to reducing opioid-related deaths in Erie County?
2. What insights about factors driving the opioid epidemic were gained by understanding its stocks, flows, and feedback loops?
3. What implications, perhaps unintended or unanticipated, will the task force interventions have in areas such as healthcare delivery or law enforcement beyond the opioid crisis?
4. How can the task force sustain achievements beyond its existence and prevent the opioid environment from reverting to a higher-mortality system?
5. How can strategies used by ECDOH for the opioid crisis be applied to other crises, such as climate change or lack of primary care access in low-income neighborhoods?

References

1. U.S. Census Bureau. (2016). QuickFacts: Erie County, New York. Retrieved from https://www.census.gov/quickfacts/fact/table/eriecountynewyork/PST045216
2. Rudd, R. A., Seth, P., David, F., & Scholl, L. (2016). Increased in drug and opioid-involved overdose deaths—United States, 2010–2015. *Morbidity and Mortality Weekly Report, 65*(50–51), 1445–1452.
3. Centers for Disease Control and Prevention. (2018). Emergency department data show rapid increased in opioid overdoses. Retrieved from https://www.cdc.gov/media/releases/2018/p0306-vs-opioids-overdoses.html

4. Moore, C. (2018). Opioid overdose prevention training [PowerPoint slides]. Erie County Opiate Task Force free community trainings. Retrieved from http://www2.erie.gov/health /index.php?q=free-community-trainings-opioid-overdose-recognition-use-naloxone-reversal

5. Tan, S. (2018, February 27). "Light at the end of the tunnel": Opioid deaths in Erie County decrease. *The Buffalo News*. Retrieved from http://www.buffalonews.com/2018/02/27/erie -county-opioid-death-rate-starting-to-fall/

6. Healy, E. (2018, February 28). Portraits in steel: The Steel Plant Museum. Retrieved from https://www.visitbuffaloniagara.com/portraits-steel-steel-plant-museum/

7. New York State Health Foundation. (2017). Targeting an epidemic: Opioid prescribing patterns by county in New York State. Retrieved from https://nyshealthfoundation.org/wp-content /uploads/2017/12/targeting-opioid-epidemic-new-york-state-dec-2017.pdf

8. New York State Department of Health. (2018). I-STOP/PMP internet system for tracking over-prescribing: Prescription monitoring program. Retrieved from https://www.health .ny.gov/professionals/narcotic/prescription_monitoring/

9. Brown, R., Riley, M. R., Ulrich, L., Kraly, E. P., Jenkins, P., Krupa, N. L., & Gadomski, A. (2017). Impact of New York prescription drug monitoring program, I-STOP, on statewide overdose morbidity. *Drug and Alcohol Dependence, 178*, 348–354.

10. Erie County Department of Health. (2018). Opiate epidemic task force. Retrieved from http:// www2.erie.gov/health/index.php?q=opiate-epidemic-task-force

11. Poloncarz, M. C. (2016). Executive order #014: Establishment of an opioid epidemic task force. Erie County Department of Health. Retrieved from http://www2.erie.gov/exec/index .php?q=executive-order-014

12. Substance Abuse and Mental Health Services Administration. (2018). SBIRT: Screening, brief intervention, and referral to treatment. Retrieved from https://www.integration.samhsa.gov /clinical-practice/sbirt

13. Thompson, C. (2017, July 9). Goal of nation's first opioid court: Keep users alive. *Associated Press*. Retrieved from https://www.usnews.com/news/news/articles/2017-07-09 /goal-of-nations-first-opioid-court-keep-users-alive

14. Plants, R. (2018, March 6). WNY hospital ERs seek ways to cut opioid ODs. *2 On Your Side*. Retrieved from https://www.wgrz.com/article/news/wny-hospital-ers-seek-ways-to -cut-opioid-ods/71-526469795

15. Senge, P. M. (2006). *The fifth discipline: The art and practice of the learning organization.* New York, NY: Crown Business.

16. Rowitz, L. (2014). *Public health leadership: Putting principles into practice.* Burlington, MA: Jones & Bartlett Learning.

Index

Page numbers followed by *f* indicate figures; those followed by *t* indicate tables.

T

U

V

W